Access your Clinics anywhere you go with our new App!

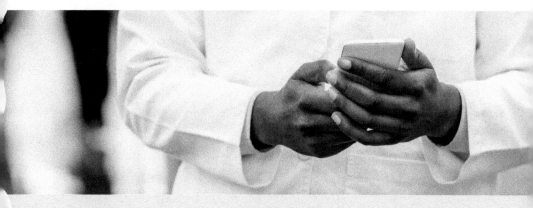

The new and improved Clinics Review Articles mobile app offers subscribers rapid access to recently published content from all Clinics Review Articles titles.

KEY FEATURES OF THE CLINICS APP:

- **Download full issues** while reading – no need to wait!
- **Access articles quickly and conveniently** with new, improved layouts and navigation.
- **Interact with figures, tables, videos**, and other supplementary content.
- **Personalize your experience** by creating reading lists and adding your own notes to articles.
- **Share your favorite articles** on social media and email useful content to colleagues.

DOWNLOAD THE CLINICS APP TODAY!

Clinics Review Articles

Technological Advances in Rehabilitation

Editors

LEROY R. LINDSAY
JOEL STEIN

PHYSICAL MEDICINE AND REHABILITATION CLINICS OF NORTH AMERICA

www.pmr.theclinics.com

Consulting Editor
SANTOS F. MARTINEZ

May 2019 • Volume 30 • Number 2

ELSEVIER

1600 John F. Kennedy Boulevard • Suite 1800 • Philadelphia, Pennsylvania, 19103-2899

http://www.theclinics.com

PHYSICAL MEDICINE AND REHABILITATION CLINICS OF NORTH AMERICA Volume 30, Number 2
May 2019 ISSN 1047-9651, ISBN 978-0-323-67780-6

Editor: Lauren Boyle
Developmental Editor: Meredith Madeira

Photocopying
Single photocopies of single articles may be made for personal use as allowed by national copyright laws. Permission of the Publisher and payment of a fee is required for all other photocopying, including multiple or systematic copying, copying for advertising or promotional purposes, resale, and all forms of document delivery. Special rates are available for educational institutions that wish to make photocopies for non-profit educational classroom use. For information on how to seek permission visit www.elsevier.com/permissions or call: (+44) 1865 843830 (UK)/(+1) 215 239 3804 (USA).

Derivative Works
Subscribers may reproduce tables of contents or prepare lists of articles including abstracts for internal circulation within their institutions. Permission of the Publisher is required for resale or distribution outside the institution. Permission of the Publisher is required for all other derivative works, including compilations and translations (please consult www.elsevier.com/permissions).

Electronic Storage or Usage
Permission of the Publisher is required to store or use electronically any material contained in this periodical, including any article or part of an article (please consult www.elsevier.com/permissions). Except as outlined above, no part of this publication may be reproduced, stored in a retrieval system or transmitted in any form or by any means, electronic, mechanical, photocopying, recording or otherwise, without prior written permission of the Publisher.

Notice
No responsibility is assumed by the Publisher for any injury and/or damage to persons or property as a matter of products liability, negligence or otherwise, or from any use or operation of any methods, products, instructions or ideas contained in the material herein. Because of rapid advances in the medical sciences, in particular, independent verification of diagnoses and drug dosages should be made.

Although all advertising material is expected to conform to ethical (medical) standards, inclusion in this publication does not constitute a guarantee or endorsement of the quality or value of such product or of the claims made of it by its manufacturer.

Reprints. For copies of 100 or more of articles in this publication, please contact the Commercial Reprints Department, Elsevier Inc., 360 Park Avenue South, New York, NY 10010-1710. Tel.: 212-633-3874; Fax: 212-633-3820; E-mail: reprints@elsevier.com.

Physical Medicine and Rehabilitation Clinics of North America (ISSN 1047-9651) is published quarterly by Elsevier Inc., 360 Park Avenue South, New York, NY 10010-1710. Months of issue are February, May, August, and November. Business and Editorial Offices: 1600 John F. Kennedy Blvd., Suite 1800, Philadelphia, PA 19103-2899. Customer Service Office: 3251 Riverport Lane, Maryland Heights, MO 63043. Periodicals postage paid at New York, NY and additional mailing offices. Subscription price per year is $304.00 (US individuals), $600.00 (US institutions), $100.00 (US students), $366.00 (Canadian individuals), $790.00 (Canadian institutions), $210.00 (Canadian students), $429.00 (foreign individuals), $790.00 (foreign institutions), and $210.00 (foreign students). Foreign air speed delivery is included in all *Clinics* subscription prices. All prices are subject to change without notice. **POSTMASTER:** Send address changes to *Physical Medicine and Rehabilitation Clinics of North America*, Customer Service Office: Elsevier Health Sciences Division, Subscription Customer Service, 3251 Riverport Lane, Maryland Heights, MO 63043. **Customer Service: 1-800-654-2452 (US). From outside of the United States, call 314-447-8871. Fax: 314-447-8029. E-mail: JournalsCustomer Service-usa@elsevier.com (for print support); JournalsOnlineSupport-usa@elsevier.com (for online support).**

Physical Medicine and Rehabilitation Clinics of North America is indexed in *Excerpta Medica, MEDLINE/ PubMed (Index Medicus), Cinahl,* and *Cumulative Index to Nursing and Allied Health Literature.*

Printed in the United States of America.

Contributors

CONSULTING EDITOR

SANTOS F. MARTINEZ, MD, MS
Diplomate of the American Academy of Physical Medicine and Rehabilitation, Certificate of Added Qualification Sports Medicine, Assistant Professor, Department of Orthopaedics, Campbell Clinic Orthopaedics, University of Tennessee, Memphis, Tennessee, USA

EDITORS

LEROY R. LINDSAY, MD
Assistant Professor of Clinical Rehabilitation Medicine, Weill Cornell Medical College, Cornell University, Adjunct Instructor in Clinical Rehabilitation Medicine, Columbia University College of Physicians and Surgeons, New York, New York, USA

JOEL STEIN, MD
Simon Baruch Professor and Chair, Department of Rehabilitation and Regenerative Medicine, Columbia University College of Physicians and Surgeons, Professor and Chair, Department of Rehabilitation Medicine, Weill Cornell Medicine, Physiatrist-in-Chief, New York-Presbyterian Hospital, New York, New York, USA

AUTHORS

SUNIL K. AGRAWAL, MSc, PhD
Professor of Mechanical Engineering and Rehabilitation/Regenerative Medicine, Columbia University, New York, New York, USA

IDRIS AMIN, MD
Department of Rehabilitation and Regenerative Medicine, Columbia University Medical Center, Department of Rehabilitation Medicine, Weill Cornell Medicine, New York, New York, USA

CLAUDIA A. ANGELI, PhD
Kentucky Spinal Cord Injury Research Center, University of Louisville, Frazier Rehab Institute, Louisville, Kentucky, USA

DENNIS BOURBEAU, PhD
MetroHealth Rehabilitation Institute, MetroHealth Medical Center, Case Western Reserve University, Cleveland FES Center, Research Service, Louis Stokes Cleveland Department of Veterans Affairs Medical Center, Cleveland, Ohio, USA

ANNE M. BRYDEN, MA, OTR/L
Cleveland FES Center, Institute for Functional Restoration, Case Western Reserve University, Cleveland, Ohio, USA

XIYA CAO, BS
PhD candidate, Mechanical Engineering, Columbia University, New York, New York, USA

JUDITH E. DEUTSCH, PT, PhD, FAPTA
Professor, Director, Rivers Lab, Department of Rehabilitation and Movement
Science, School of Health Professions, Rutgers University, Newark,
New Jersey, USA

ANTHONY F. DIMARCO, MD
MetroHealth Rehabilitation Institute, MetroHealth Medical Center, Professor, Physical
Medicine and Rehabilitation, Physiology and Biophysics, Institute for Functional
Restoration, Case Western Reserve University, Cleveland FES Center, Cleveland,
Ohio, USA

ALBERTO ESQUENAZI, MD
Director, MossRehab Gait and Motion Analysis Laboratory, Professor of Physical
Medicine and Rehabilitation, Elkins Park, Pennsylvania, USA

STEVE R. FISHER, PT, PhD, GCS
Associate Professor, Department of Physical Therapy, The University of Texas Medical
Branch, Galveston, Texas, USA

GERARD E. FRANCISCO, MD
Professor, Department of Physical Medicine and Rehabilitation, McGovern Medical
School, The University of Texas Health Science Center at Houston, NeuroRecovery
Research Center at TIRR Memorial Hermann, Houston, Texas, USA

MARINELLA DᴇFRE GALEA, MD
Chief, Department of Spinal Cord Injury and Disorder, Director, Amyotrophic Lateral
Sclerosis Program, Co-Director, Multiple Sclerosis Regional Center, The James J. Peters
VA Medical Center, Bronx, New York, USA; Assistant Professor, Department of Physical
Medicine and Rehabilitation, Icahn School of Medicine at Mount Sinai, Assistant
Professor, Columbia University, School of Medicine, New York, New York, USA

ALFRED C. GELLHORN, MD
Department of Rehabilitation Medicine, Weill Cornell Medicine, New York, New York, USA

ANDREW M. GORDON, PhD
Professor, Department of Biobehavioral Sciences, Teachers College, Columbia
University, New York, New York, USA

JAMES E. GRAHAM, PhD, DC
Professor, Department of Occupational Therapy, Director, Center for Community
Partnerships, Colorado State University, Fort Collins, Colorado, USA

STEPHEN HAMPTON, MD
Assistant Professor, Department of Physical Medicine and Rehabilitation, University of
Pennsylvania, Perelman School of Medicine, Philadelphia, Pennsylvania, USA

RICHARD L. HARVEY, MD
Department of Physical Medicine and Rehabilitation, Feinberg School of Medicine,
Northwestern University, Clinical Chair, Brain Innovation Center, Shirley Ryan AbilityLab,
Chicago, Illinois, USA

JEFFREY T. HECKMAN, DO
Medical Director, VA Amputation System of Care Regional Amputation Center, Division of
Rehabilitation Care Services, VA Puget Sound Health Care System, Associate Professor,
Department of Rehabilitation Medicine, University of Washington, Seattle, Washington,
USA

JULIO C. HERNANDEZ-PAVON, PhD, DSc
Department of Physical Medicine and Rehabilitation, Feinberg School of Medicine, Northwestern University, Center for Brain Stimulation, Shirley Ryan AbilityLab, Chicago, Illinois, USA

BRITTANY HOEHLEIN, SDPT
Research Assistant, Rivers Lab, Department of Rehabilitation and Movement Science, School of Health Professions, Rutgers University, Newark, New Jersey, USA

SHANNON JUENGST, PhD, CRC
Assistant Professor, Department of Physical Medicine and Rehabilitation, The University of Texas Southwestern Medical Center, Dallas, Texas, USA

DONALD KASITINON, MD
Department of Physical Medicine and Rehabilitation, The University of Texas Southwestern Medical Center, Dallas, Texas, USA

G. ELI KAUFMAN, CPO
Division of Rehabilitation Care Services, VA Puget Sound Health Care System, Center for Limb Loss and Mobility (CLiMB), Department of Veterans Affairs, Office of Research and Development, Seattle, Washington, USA

MARY S. KESZLER, MD
Division of Rehabilitation Care Services, VA Puget Sound Health Care System, Department of Rehabilitation Medicine, University of Washington, Seattle, Washington, USA

KEVIN L. KILGORE, PhD
MetroHealth Rehabilitation Institute, Departments of Orthopaedics and Physical Medicine and Rehabilitation, MetroHealth Medical Center, Case Western Reserve University, Cleveland FES Center, Research Service, Louis Stokes Cleveland Department of Veterans Affairs Medical Center, Cleveland, Ohio, USA

JAYME S. KNUTSON, PhD
Director of Research, MetroHealth Rehabilitation Institute, MetroHealth Medical Center, Associate Professor, Case Western Reserve University, Cleveland FES Center, Research Service, Louis Stokes Cleveland Department of Veterans Affairs Medical Center, Cleveland, Ohio, USA

KRZYSZTOF E. KOWALSKI, PhD
Clinical Associate Professor of Medicine, Case Western Reserve University, Cleveland FES Center, Research Service, Louis Stokes Cleveland Department of Veterans Affairs Medical Center, Department of Medicine, MetroHealth Medical Center, Cleveland, Ohio, USA

NATHANIEL MAKOWSKI, PhD
MetroHealth Rehabilitation Institute, MetroHealth Medical Center, Case Western Reserve University, Cleveland FES Center, Cleveland, Ohio, USA

DAVID C. MORGENROTH, MD
Division of Rehabilitation Care Services, VA Puget Sound Health Care System, Associate Professor, Department of Rehabilitation Medicine, University of Washington, Investigator, Center for Limb Loss and Mobility (CLiMB), Department of Veterans Affairs, Office of Research and Development, Seattle, Washington, USA

CANDICE OSBORNE, PhD, MPH, OTR
Assistant Professor, Department of Physical Medicine and Rehabilitation, The University of Texas Southwestern Medical Center, Dallas, Texas, USA

KENNETH J. OTTENBACHER, PhD, OTR
Professor and Director, Division of Rehabilitation Sciences, The University of Texas Medical Branch, Galveston, Texas, USA

ANTONIO PRADO, BS, MSc
PhD candidate, Mechanical Engineering, Columbia University, New York, New York, USA

URŠKA PUH, PT, PhD
Assistant Professor, Department of Physiotherapy, Faculty of Health Sciences, University of Ljubljana, Ljubljana, Slovenia

LINDSAY RAMEY, MD
Assistant Professor, Department of Physical Medicine and Rehabilitation, The University of Texas Southwestern Medical Center, Dallas, Texas, USA

ENRICO REJC, PhD
Kentucky Spinal Cord Injury Research Center, Department of Neurological Surgery, University of Louisville, Louisville, Kentucky, USA

MAXIME T. ROBERT, MSc, PhD
Postdoctoral Research Fellow, Department of Biobehavioral Sciences, Teachers College, Columbia University, New York, New York, USA

MUKUL TALATY, PhD
MossRehab Gait and Motion Analysis Laboratory, Elkins Park, Pennsylvania, USA

RICHARD D. WILSON, MD, MS
Director, Division of Neurologic Rehabilitation, MetroHealth Rehabilitation Institute, MetroHealth Medical Center, Associate Professor of Physical Medicine and Rehabilitation, Case Western Reserve University, Cleveland FES Center, Cleveland, Ohio, USA

NURAY YOZBATIRAN, PT, PhD
Assistant Professor, Department of Physical Medicine and Rehabilitation, McGovern Medical School, The University of Texas Health Science Center at Houston, NeuroRecovery Research Center at TIRR Memorial Hermann, Houston, Texas, USA

Contents

stimulation technology are needed to better understand the recovery potential in this population.

The authors present a Recurrent Neural Network classifier model that segments the walking data recorded with instrumented footwear. The signals from 3 piezoresistive sensors, a 3-axis accelerometer, and Euler angles are used to generate temporal gait characteristics of a user. The model was tested using a data set collected from 28 adults containing 4198 steps. The mean errors for heel strikes and toe-offs were -5.9 ± 37.1 and 11.4 ± 47.4 milliseconds. These small errors show that the algorithm can be reliably used to segment the gait recordings and to use this segmentation to estimate temporal parameters of the subjects.

Tetraplegia resulting from cervical injury is the most frequent neurologic category after spinal cord injury and causes substantial disability. The residual strength of partially paralyzed muscles is an important determinant of independence and function in tetraplegia. Small improvements in upper extremity function can make a clinically significant difference in daily activities. Major advances in rehabilitation technologies over the past 2 decades have allowed testing of robotic devices in rehabilitation of motor impairments. This literature assessment provides an overview of robotic-assisted training research for improving arm and hand functions after cervical spinal cord injury.

Improving walking function is a desirable outcome in rehabilitation and of high importance for social and vocational reintegration for persons with neurologic-related gait impairment. Robots for lower limb gait rehabilitation are designed principally to help automate repetitive labor-intensive training during neurorehabilitation. These include tethered exoskeletons, end-effector devices, untethered exoskeletons, and patient-guided suspension systems. This article reviews the first 3 categories and briefly mentions the fourth. Research is needed to further define the therapeutic applications of these devices. Additional technical improvements are expected regarding device size, controls, and battery life for untethered devices.

The validity and reliability of using the Kinect camera to measure standardized assessment of transitional movement, stepping, and balance was systematically reviewed and critically appraised for quality of the methods and results. The study made recommendations of specific tests for practice based on inclusion of both validity and reliability testing as well as quality of results. Authors' willingness to share their software was reported. Translation into practice is limited by lack of redundancy among studies and access to the software to implement the tests.

Amputation results in a wide range of functional limitations; advances in surgical, rehabilitative, and prosthetic care are aimed at optimizing functional quality of life for the spectrum of individuals with limb loss. This article initially focuses on advances in surgical and rehabilitative care, followed by noteworthy advances in prosthetics, including potential advantages and disadvantages. Although prosthetics tend to dominate attention in the field, it is important to remember that optimizing surgical and rehabilitative care are vital components of enhancing functional recovery and quality of life in people with limb loss.

Platelet-rich plasma (PRP) is a novel therapeutic treatment option for joint and tendon disease, but preparation methods are varied. This article summarizes research on uses of PRP, compares classification systems to standardize various PRP compositions, and discusses the most common methodologies to produce PRP. Even with advances in understanding PRP, there are unknowns about the factors and processes that may have an impact on treatment efficacy for musculoskeletal conditions. PRP studies should pursue determining optimal PRP preparation, setting a standard to evaluate PRP mixtures and preparation methods, assessing efficacy of PRP for various musculoskeletal conditions, and managing and reducing costs.

Recent advances in commercial home automation, or Smart Home, technology may augment adaptive living. Although these interconnected devices were not designed specifically for individuals with disabilities, they may increase independence with tasks in the home, such as adjusting the temperature or lighting, cleaning, and maintaining home security. As these integrated systems continue to advance in capability and availability, the potential for adaptive application continues to grow. This article highlights categories of currently available consumer devices with potential for application to adaptive living, and outlines the ways in which these novel devices might augment more traditional approaches to maximizing function.

The biomedical scientific community is in the midst of a significant expansion in how data are used to accomplish the important goals of reducing disability and improving health care. Data science is the academic discipline emerging from this expansion. Data science reflects a new approach to the acquisition, storage, analysis, and interpretation of scientific knowledge. The potential benefits of data science are transforming biomedical research and will lead physical medicine and rehabilitation in exciting new directions. Understanding this transformation will require modifying and expanding the education, training, and research infrastructure that support rehabilitation science and practice.

Telerehabilitation refers to the virtual delivery of rehabilitation services into the patient's home. This methodology has shown to be advantageous when used to enhance or replace conventional therapy to overcome geographic, physical, and cognitive barriers. The exponential growth of technology has led to the development of new applications that enable health care providers to monitor, educate, treat, and support patients in their own environment. Best practices and well-designed Telerehabilitation studies are needed to build and sustain a strong Telerehabilitation system that is integrated in the current health care structure and is cost-effective.

Although there is disparity in access to mobile health (mHealth) services among people with disabilities, several smartphone and tablet-based mHealth applications are available that may affect the care of patients in rehabilitation medicine. This article reviews the current evidence for and breadth of application-based mHealth interventions in rehabilitation medicine, including comprehensive self-management mHealth services; weight management mHealth services; diagnosis-specific mHealth services for individuals with brain, spinal cord, musculoskeletal, or other injury types; and nonmedical services to improve community and social integration.

PHYSICAL MEDICINE AND REHABILITATION CLINICS OF NORTH AMERICA

SERIES OF RELATED INTEREST

Orthopedic Clinics
Clinics in Sports Medicine

VISIT THE CLINICS ONLINE!
Access your subscription at:
www.theclinics.com

Foreword

It Is a New Beginning

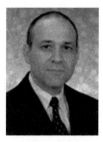

Santos F. Martinez, MD, MS
Consulting Editor

I would like to thank Dr Stein and Dr Lindsay for taking on this issue. The momentum for innovation is fertile with evermore diversity in approaches to address obstacles and limitations frequently encountered in the rehabilitation population. It is hoped that such advances will take us past preconceived limitations accessing technology, which will enrich the quality of life of our patients and thus our society. This issue also provokes a reassessment of our daily clinical practices, where innovation will and is allowing remote interaction with practitioners, patients, and devices. Provided we maintain focus, the future holds great promise, where impairments and disabilities will be perceived with less reservation. Technological advances with a growth in regenerative medicine, nanotechnology, artificial intelligence, alternative frontiers with neurocognitive, and orthotic/prosthetic approaches will redefine the norm.

Santos F. Martinez, MD, MS
American Academy of Physical Medicine and Rehabilitation
Campbell Clinic Orthopaedics
Department of Orthopaedics
University of Tennessee
Memphis, TN 38104, USA

E-mail address:
smartinez@campbellclinic.com

1047-9651/19/© 2019 Published by Elsevier Inc.

Preface

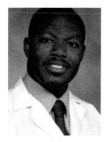 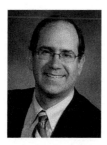

Leroy R. Lindsay, MD   Joel Stein, MD
Editors

This issue of *Physical Medicine and Rehabilitation Clinics of North America* explores the relationship between technological advances and their current and future applications in the world of rehabilitation medicine. This issue came about through discussions with students, colleagues, and mentors about future directions in various rehabilitation medicine subspecialties. While there are many forums to learn about new technologies, the number that is attempting to address possible research opportunities and use in rehabilitation is few. This issue is directed at the clinician/scientist at any stage in training.

Since the beginnings of rehabilitation medicine, technological advances and clinical applications have been intertwined. Many of the technologies being developed and adopted today have their roots in the past, including prostheses, mobility devices, neuromodulation, and robotic-based exercise therapies. New technologies have been a major driver of improved care in our specialty. Indeed, rehabilitation practitioners have used everything from physical modalities to the mastery of simple machines to treat pain and improve function and quality of life for this unique patient population. This issue is unique in that it attempts to highlight a few key areas that are particularly exciting and representative of the direction of the field as a whole.

This issue of *Physical Medicine and Rehabilitation Clinics of North America* is divided into 13 articles that span the gamut from updates on the use of robotics in rehabilitation to the basic science behind outpatient regenerative interventions. An example of an exciting development is in the area of telemedicine; this will deliver rehabilitative services to the patient at home while minimizing barriers to care. In addition, use of smart device technologies and applications is growing and highlighting the need for health provider involvement in product development, research design, and content.

While this issue is by no means a definitive summary of all that is happening in the rehabilitation and technological space, we hope that it provides an intriguing and

Phys Med Rehabil Clin N Am 30 (2019) xv–xvi
https://doi.org/10.1016/j.pmr.2019.02.001
1047-9651/19/© 2019 Published by Elsevier Inc.

encouraging summary. By highlighting these spaces for future basic science and clinical research, we hope to strengthen the field as we move into an ever-changing future.

Leroy R. Lindsay, MD
Department of Rehabilitation Medicine
Weill Cornell Medicine
New York-Presbyterian Hospital
525 E68th Street
New York, NY 10065, USA

Joel Stein, MD
Department of Rehabilitation and
Regenerative Medicine
Columbia University College of
Physicians and Surgeons
Department of Rehabilitation Medicine
Weill Cornell Medicine
New York-Presbyterian Hospital
180 Fort Washington Avenue
New York, NY 10032, USA

E-mail addresses:
lel9053@med.cornell.edu (L.R. Lindsay)
js1165@cumc.columbia.edu (J. Stein)

Neuromodulation for Functional Electrical Stimulation

Richard D. Wilson, MD, MS[a,b,c,*], Anne M. Bryden, MA, OTR/L[b,c,d,1],
Kevin L. Kilgore, PhD[a,b,c,e,f,1], Nathaniel Makowski, PhD[a,b,c,1],
Dennis Bourbeau, PhD[a,b,c,f,1], Krzysztof E. Kowalski, PhD[b,c,f,g,2],
Anthony F. DiMarco, MD[a,c,d,2], Jayme S. Knutson, PhD[a,b,c,f,1]

KEYWORDS

- Rehabilitation • Electrical stimulation • Stroke • Spinal cord injury

KEY POINTS

- Neuromodulation for functional rehabilitation uses electrical stimulation to generate or suppress activity in the nervous system in those who have suffered neurologic damage.
- Technological advances and greater understanding of the structure and function of the nervous system have enabled bioengineers and clinicians to develop treatments and devices to improve the health, function, and quality of life of those with disabilities.
- Specific applications for individuals with spinal cord injury include use as a neuroprosthesis for paralysis, to improve neurogenic bladder, and to improve lost respiratory function.
- Specific applications in stroke include electrical stimulation as a treatment to improve motor recovery and as a neuroprosthesis in the lower limb.
- Some of the devices and treatments are commercially available and some remain in the experimental realm.

Disclosure Statement: Dr A.F. DiMarco is a shareholder in Synapse biomedical, a manufacturer of diaphragm pacing systems. He holds patents on the use of spinal cord stimulation to restore cough. Dr J.S. Knutson is an inventor on U.S. Patent 8,165,685 describing contralaterally controlled functional electrical stimulation. Drs R.D. Wilson, A.M. Bryden, K.L. Kilgore, N. Makowski, D. Bourbeau, and K.E. Kowalski have nothing to disclose.
^a MetroHealth Rehabilitation Institute, MetroHealth Medical Center, Cleveland, OH, USA;
^b Case Western Reserve University, Cleveland, OH, USA; ^c Cleveland FES Center, Cleveland, OH, USA; ^d Institute for Functional Restoration, Case Western Reserve University, Cleveland, OH, USA; ^e Department of Orthopaedics, MetroHealth Medical Center, Cleveland, OH, USA; ^f Research Service, Louis Stokes Cleveland Department of Veterans Affairs Medical Center, Cleveland, OH, USA; ^g Department of Medicine, MetroHealth Medical Center, Cleveland, OH, USA
¹ Present address: 4229 Pearl Road, Cleveland, OH 44109.
² Present address: 2500 MetroHealth Drive, Cleveland, OH 44109.
* Corresponding author. 4229 Pearl Road, Cleveland, OH 44109.
E-mail address: rwilson@metrohealth.org

NEUROMODULATION TO IMPROVE FUNCTION IN SPINAL CORD INJURY

Applications of electrical stimulation are among the most promising methods for neuromodulation to provide significant gain in function for people living with spinal cord injury (SCI). SCI is a condition where people experience a gradient of functional deficits, depending on the level and severity of the lesion. Individuals with higher cervical–level injury desire restoration of upper limb function, postural stability, and respiratory function, such as the ability to cough, whereas individuals with lower lesions desire restoration of postural stability and lower limb function. Nearly all individuals living with SCI desire improvements in bladder, bowel, and sexual functions.[1] The application of electrical stimulation as a neuroprosthesis can provide such functional benefits.

A Networked Neuroprosthesis to Restore Motor Function

Neuroprostheses have been used for functional restoration in SCI. In general, electrically stimulated paralyzed muscles are activated in coordinated patterns to produce functional movements, such as grasping or stepping. Neuroprosthetic users are given control over the stimulated patterns using their residual voluntary function. Existing neuroprosthetic systems include those for bladder,[2] breathing,[3,4] cough,[5] grasp,[6,7] reaching,[8] posture control,[9,10] standing,[10,11] and walking.[12,13] These systems have been shown to provide functional benefits that cannot be gained through other interventions.[14]

The latest innovation in implanted neuroprostheses for people with SCI consists of a fully implanted system designed to restore multiple functions with a single system. The networked neuroprosthesis (NNP) can stimulate paralyzed muscles throughout the body and record myoelectric signals from muscles under voluntary control (**Fig. 1**). Coordinated stimulation patterns can be programmed into the NNP to create functional movements on command. This system can provide individuals who have motor complete cervical SCI with grasp opening and closing, overhead reach, and postural stability. The addition of cough and bladder function is anticipated. The NNP system also includes continuous temperature monitoring and 3-axis accelerometer data to record torso and upper extremity motion. The results have been positive, and demonstrated activities include eating with a fork, writing, and getting items out of a refrigerator.

Neuromodulation to Improve Bladder Function

The bladder has 2 main functions—storage of urine with continence and emptying or voiding at a chosen time and place. After SCI, most individuals develop neurogenic bladder dysfunction, which is typified by aberrant reflexes resulting in neurogenic detrusor overactivity (NDO) and often detrusor-sphincter dyssynergia. NDO, where the bladder reflexively contracts at small bladder volumes, can result in urinary incontinence, ureteral reflux, and renal damage and can trigger autonomic dysreflexia. Detrusor-sphincter dyssynergia, where the urethral sphincter simultaneously contracts at the same time as detrusor contraction, can result in inefficient or incomplete voiding. Neurogenic bladder dysfunction has a significant and adverse effect on health and quality of life. Complications from managing the neurogenic bladder, such as urinary tract infections, account for a majority of rehospitalizations after the initial injury.[15] Individuals with SCI prioritize bladder control highly[1] and there remains an unmet need for restoring bladder function after SCI.

Electrical stimulation to improve urine storage can be achieved by modulating reflex pathways that result in inhibition of unwanted bladder activity. Sacral neuromodulation (SNM) involves stimulation via a single electrode lead typically placed in the extradural

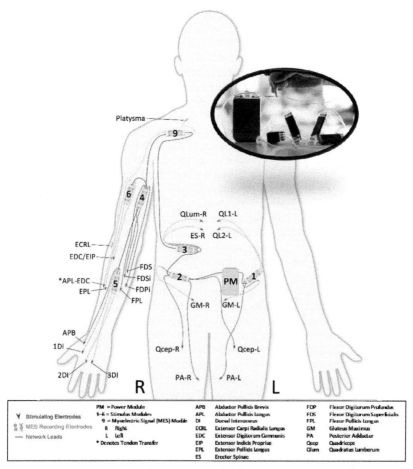

Fig. 1. Example configuration of the NNP for providing hand grasp, reach, and posture control in a single individual. NNP components consist of stimulating and recording modules (numbered 1–9), a power module, stimulating electrodes, recording electrodes, and network cables. This system consists of 24 stimulating electrodes, located as shown, and 2 myoelectric signal recording electrodes. (*Courtesy of* Kevin Kilgore, PhD, Case Western Reserve University School of Medicine and MetroHealth Medical Center, Cleveland, OH.)

space at sacral root S2, which activates sensory afferents in the posterior sacral root and is believed to modulate a bladder inhibitory reflex.[16] The implantable InterStim device (Medtronic, Minneapolis, Minnesota) has been approved for treating overactive bladder in neurologically intact individuals. Posterior tibial nerve stimulation is similarly approved for treating overactive bladder and is generally performed as an outpatient procedure approximately once per week for at least 12 sessions using a device, such as the Urgent PC (Uroplasty, Minnetonka, Minnesota).[17] Although both SNM and posterior tibial nerve stimulation are effective for improving urinary continence in individuals with overactive bladder, there are few data on the effectiveness of these approaches for individuals with NDO. There is some evidence, however, that introducing SNM in the early period after SCI may improve urinary continence for individuals with NDO.[18]

Genital nerve stimulation is an approach that can strongly inhibit bladder activity for individuals with NDO.[19] Preclinical experiments suggest that activation of the sensory afferents in the genital nerve branch of the pudendal nerves modulates a spinal reflex pathway that inhibits bladder activity by increasing sympathetic activity in the hypogastric nerve. Human testing from multiple groups have shown significant acute improvements in bladder capacity and urinary continence, and there is growing evidence for chronic feasibility and effectiveness in human subjects.[20,21] The genital nerve is close to the skin surface and can be stimulated with noninvasive surface electrodes without discomfort. Because the genital nerve contains only sensory afferents, higher stimulation amplitudes can be used without directly evoking motor responses. There is not a clinically available product available for this approach, but genital nerve stimulation could become another option for improving bladder control after SCI.

Sacral anterior root stimulation (SARS) has shown efficient bladder emptying for individuals with SCI.[22] The Finetech-Brindley – Bladder Control System (Finetech Medical Ltd., Welwyn Garden City, Hertfordshire, UK) is currently available but not in all countries. This system involves an external stimulator and controller that communicate wirelessly through the skin to electrodes implanted at the sacral roots to stimulate the nerves that control the bladder. The preganglionic parasympathetic nerve fibers that drive detrusor activity pass through the anterior sacral spinal roots. SARS takes advantage of this central, stable location for electrically stimulating these motor neurons to evoke contractions of the bladder wall. This approach is appropriate for individuals with an upper motor neuron lesion whose preganglionic nerve pathways to the bladder remain intact. The anterior roots also include the motor efferents for other structures, such as the urethral sphincter. The co-contractions of the urethral sphincter and detrusor muscle evoked by SARS can impede bladder emptying. To address this issue, stimulation strategies take advantage of the urethral sphincter muscle relaxing quickly after the cessation of stimulation whereas the detrusor muscle relaxes much more slowly. Stimulation can be delivered as a train of pulses in quick succession, causing both the urethral sphincter and detrusor to contract. When stimulation ceases, the sphincter relaxes almost instantly while the detrusor slowly relaxes and maintains intravesicular pressure for voiding. Bladder emptying is achieved between bursts of stimulation. This process is usually repeated several times to completely empty the bladder.

There are challenges with SARS that reduce adoption in the SCI community. First, it requires an invasive surgical procedure in which a laminectomy is performed to expose the sacral roots for electrode implantation. A posterior rhizotomy of the sacral roots is also performed to inhibit unwanted urethral sphincter reflexes that can prevent efficient bladder emptying.[22] The posterior rhizotomy causes a loss of pelvic sensation and desirable reflexes, including reflex sexual functions, such as erection. This issue is particularly important because most individuals with SCI have an incomplete lesion and may retain some function and sensation below the lesion level.

To overcome the challenges associated with the posterior rhizotomy, alternative patterns of electrical stimulation are being tested, including kilohertz high-frequency stimulation. Kilohertz high-frequency stimulation has the potential to block conduction of action potentials in the sacral roots, which could be as effective as transecting them. The benefits of this high-frequency approach are that it is available on demand and it is completely reversible. Kilohertz high-frequency stimulation of the sacral roots has undergone preclinical testing and has been shown to inhibit urethral sphincter activity and improve bladder emptying.[23] Another alternative to the posterior rhizotomy for controlling NDO is to modify SNM, described previously, by administering low-frequency stimulation at multiple sacral roots, rather than just 1, targeting all the sensory afferents that pass through the pudendal nerve.

Neuromodulation to Improve Pulmonary Function

Patients with high thoracic SCI suffer from paralysis of the major portion of both their inspiratory and expiratory muscles. Loss of inspiratory muscle function, including the diaphragm, results in respiratory failure requiring lifelong ventilatory support. Loss of expiratory muscle function severely limits the capacity of these patients to cough and expel secretions, resulting in a high incidence of respiratory tract infections. Neuromodulation with electrical stimulation can be used to restore respiratory function so that those with respiratory failure can be liberated from mechanical ventilation (MV).

The diaphragm is the major muscle of inspiration and is enervated by the phrenic nerves that arise from the cervical spinal nerves C3, C4, and C5. Patients with lower cervical SCI and preserved phrenic nerve function can breathe comfortably without assistance. Loss of phrenic nerve function typically results in respiratory failure. MV is a life-saving measure to support ventilation in patients with acute respiratory failure secondary to SCI. In the United States alone, as many as 400 to 500 new patients each year require MV.[24] Diaphragm pacing (DP) is an alternative to MV, with significant advantages, including improved sense of well-being and overall health (**Box 1**).[25] The basic design of currently available DP systems is similar, with each device requiring bilateral stimulation of the phrenic nerves (**Fig. 2**).

Success of the DP is dependent on the integrity of the phrenic nerves. The Mark IV Diaphragm Pacemaker System (Avery Biomedical Devices, Commack, New York) requires the placement of electrodes directly on the phrenic nerves in the thorax.[26] Wires are tunneled subcutaneously to connect the electrodes to radiofrequency receivers that are positioned over the anterior chest wall. Radiofrequency signals are generated by an external battery–powered transmitter, which is inductively coupled to the receivers via circular rubberized antennas. A similar device is the Atrostim PNS V2.0

Box 1
Potential benefits of diaphragmatic pacing

Increased mobility
   Easier transfers from bed to chair
   Easier transport to occupational and recreational activities outside of the home

Restoration of olfactory sensation

Improved speech

Subjective sense of more normal breathing
   Engagement of intrinsic respiratory muscles
   Normal negative-pressure ventilation

Reduced anxiety and embarrassment
   Elimination of ventilator tubing
   Elimination of ventilator noise
   Daytime closure of tracheostomy

Improved level of comfort
   Elimination of fear of ventilator disconnection
   Elimination of the pull of ventilator tubing
   Elimination of the discomfort associated with positive-pressure breathing

Reduction in the incidence of respiratory tract infections

Reduction in overall costs
   Reduction and/or elimination of ventilator supplies
   Reduction in the level of required caregiver support

From DiMarco AF. Diaphram pacing. Clin Chest Med 2018;39:2; with permission.

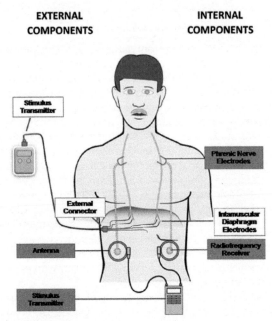

Fig. 2. Components of diaphragmatic pacing systems. (*From* DiMarco AF. Diaphram pacing. Clin Chest Med 2018;39:2; with permission.)

(Atrotech, Tampere, Finland) but is not available in the United States. DP can also be achieved by placement of electrodes within the diaphragm near the phrenic nerve motor points bilaterally with use of the NeuRx RA/4 device (Synapse Biomedical, Oberlin, Ohio). Although electrodes are positioned within the diaphragm, success of this technique is still dependent on phrenic nerve stimulation and, therefore, represents another method of phrenic nerve pacing. These electrodes can be placed via minimally invasive laparascopic surgery and without the risk of phrenic nerve injury because the electrodes are not placed directly on the phrenic nerves. In patients with phrenic nerve injury, intercostal to phrenic nerve transfer holds promise as an alternative method of DP.[27]

Clinical studies have demonstrated that DP is both an efficacious and a cost-effective method of providing ventilatory support in patients with SCI. As many as 50% of patients who are dependent on tracheostomy MV are able to use DP as the sole method of ventilatory support.[3,28] Effective DP requires an intact phrenic nerve to allow the muscle to be stimulated to provide adequate ventilation and a healthy diaphragm muscle. There are several reasons why DP may not be successful in maintaining full-time ventilatory support. First, peripheral nerve electrodes typically do not achieve complete diaphragm activation due to the high activation thresholds of some axons. Second, due to conditioning of the diaphragm with use from chronic low-frequency electrical stimulation, conversion of the diaphragm back to efficient type I muscle increases endurance but reduces maximum force generation and thereby reduces inspiratory volume. Finally, the diaphragm accounts for approximately 60% of the inspiratory capacity. Lack of participation of the intercostal muscles, therefore, may also result in insufficient inspiratory volume. The incidence of complications and side effects associated with DP is low but may include iatrogenic injury to the phrenic nerve, technical malfunction of the external and implanted components, and infection.[29]

Future developments in animal models suggest the both the diaphragm and intercostal muscles can be activated in synchrony by the application of high-frequency upper thoracic spinal cord stimulation (SCS).[30] Clinical trials of this technique are necessary to assess its safety and efficacy.

Patients with SCI may have impaired cough and difficulty expelling secretions due to expiratory muscle paralysis, contributing to the high incidence of respiratory tract infections and associated morbidity and mortality. Current modalities in clinical practice include gravity, active suctioning with a catheter, manually assisted coughing whereby external force is applied to the abdominal wall, and use of a mechanical insufflation-exsufflation device.[31] Although each of these methods has shown some efficacy, they are often uncomfortable and labor intensive and require specialized equipment and provider-patient coordination. Neuromodulation can provide an alternative means to restore effective cough.

A normal cough is characterized by an explosive expiration that provides a protective mechanism to clear the airway of secretions and foreign material. The cough reflex is composed of several phases that occur in sequence (**Fig. 3**). The initial phase consists of a variable-sized inspiration, which is followed by glottic closure and then expiratory muscle contraction, which results in the development of large intrathoracic pressures.[32] In the final phase, the vocal cords and epiglottis open widely, resulting in the development of rapid airflow rates that cause expectoration of foreign bodies or secretions from the airway. Experimental methods have been proposed to activate the expiratory muscles, including magnetic stimulation,[32] surface abdominal stimulation,[33] and SCS.[5] The largest clinical experience has been achieved with SCS.

SCS to restore cough has been achieved using a fully implantable electrical stimulation system (Finetech Medical, Welwyn Garden City, United Kingdom) that requires laminotomies to place 3 single-disk electrodes in the dorsal epidural space at the T9, T11, and L1 spinal levels (**Fig. 4**).[5] The effects of lower thoracic SCS on airway pressure and peak airflow rates at different spinal levels is shown for 1 subject in **Fig. 5A, B**.

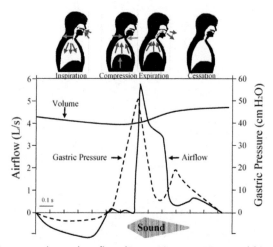

Fig. 3. Phases of a normal cough reflex. (*From* Dimarco AF, Kowalski KE. Restoration of Cough via Functional Electrical Stimulation. In: Krames ES, Peckham PH, Rezai AR, Eds. Neuromodulation: comprehensive textbook of principles, technologies, and therapies. 2nd Ed. London, England; 2018:1355-1370; with permission.)

Neuromodulation to restore cough reduces the need for suctioning/assisted cough, improves the ease in raising sputum, and can eliminate the need for the use of other means of secretion clearance. In the initial group of subjects, the need for caregiver support to manage secretions (**Fig. 5C**) and, importantly, the incidence of respiratory tract infections fell significantly (**Fig. 5D**).

The complications and side effects associated with implantation of this system were infrequent and typically mild. Approximately 30% of patients developed signs of autonomic dysfunction, including elevations in blood pressure and reductions in heart rate, which were asymptomatic. These changes resolved within 5 minutes to 10 minutes after discontinuation of SCS. After chronic daily stimulation, these changes gradually diminished in frequency and severity and disappeared completely within weeks with frequent use of the device. Some patients developed mild contraction of the lower limbs, which was eliminated by reduction in stimulus parameters. There was no evidence of bowel or bladder leakage.

Despite the substantial cost of the device, and costs associated with surgical implantation, a cost-benefit analysis of use of the cough system demonstrated a marked reduction in the overall costs of respiratory care, such that a break-even point was achieved in the first year after implantation.[34]

NEUROMODULATION TO IMPROVE FUNCTION IN STROKE
Neuromodulation for Upper Limb Motor Relearning

The most common upper limb motor impairments targeted for neuromuscular electrical stimulation (NMES) treatment in stroke survivors are inability and decreased ability

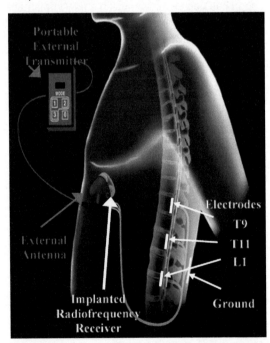

Fig. 4. Fully implantable electrical stimulation system for SCS to restore cough. (*From* Dimarco AF, Kowalski KE. Restoration of Cough via Functional Electrical Stimulation. In: Krames ES, Peckham PH, Rezai AR, Eds. Neuromodulation: comprehensive textbook of principles, technologies, and therapies. 2nd Ed. London, England; 2018:1355-1370; with permission.)

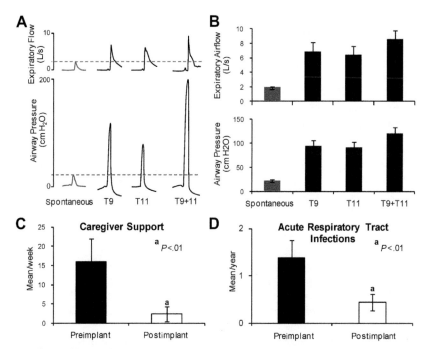

Fig. 5. Effects of lower thoracic neuromodulation to restore cough in SCI: (*A, B*) airway pressure and peak airflow with stimulation at different spinal levels; (*C*) reduction in caregiver support; and (*D*) reduction in acute respiratory tract infections. (*Courtesy of* the American Thoracic Society, New York. Copyright 2018 American Thoracic Society; with permission.)

to volitionally extend the elbow, wrist, and finger and thumb. These impairments have a profound impact on stroke survivors' function, participation, and quality of life. The purpose of most upper limb stroke NMES applications is to produce a persistent therapeutic effect, that is, improve recovery of volitional upper limb function. Therefore, these applications are temporary and noninvasive, with surface electrodes typically placed over the paretic finger and wrist muscles. Elbow extensors and/or shoulder muscles also may be targeted in some applications.

Although the mechanisms of action of NMES are not completely understood, there is evidence that NMES may improve strength, active range of motion, coordination, and/or motor control via peripheral or central mechanisms or both. Central effects of NMES also may contribute to functional improvement. There is emerging evidence of both peripheral and central effects that are likely to be dependent on severity of central nervous system damage caused by the stroke and time poststroke, factors that have been found important predictors of poststroke improvement.[35,36]

NMES that is delivered according to the timing and intensity settings of the stimulator is called cyclic NMES. Cyclic NMES turns on for several seconds and then turns off for several seconds, repeating the cycle for as long as the device is on.[37] The device does not require a patient to contribute any simultaneous effort to move the arm or hand. For patients who have a high degree of spasticity that increases with attempts to move the upper limb, cyclic NMES may be most appropriate because the participant can remain relaxed during the stimulation.

Button switch–triggered NMES allows a user[38] or therapist[39] to control the timing of the stimulation by pressing button switches on the device. For example, 1 button press may turn on stimulation to the finger and thumb extensors to provide an open hand. Another button press may turn off stimulation to the finger and thumb extensors. This control of the timing makes it possible to use the stimulator as an assistive device during task practice,[38] an advantage over cyclic NMES. Incorporating NMES into task practice is believed to be a way of enhancing the effect of task practice without the assistance of NMES. With button switch–triggered NMES devices, the intensity of stimulation (ie, pulse amplitude, frequency, and duration) are typically preset to levels that produce strong muscle contractions and desired arm or hand movement without pain.

Sensors worn on a patient's body may be a means of giving patients a greater sense of control of the stimulation and, therefore, the affected limb. For example, electromyogram (EMG)-triggered NMES uses EMG recording electrodes over the paretic wrist muscles to detect even weak attempts to extend the wrist and/or open the hand.[40] If the detected EMG signal exceeds a certain minimum threshold set by the therapist, then the stimulator turns on and produces wrist extension and hand opening. The pairing of motor intention, the stimulated response, and the corresponding proprioceptive feedback to the brain may have central effects that help restore neural circuits necessary for recovery of volitional movement and function.[41] Other body-worn sensors, such as accelerometers, may make it possible to deliver stimulation with timing that is even more seamless and synergistic with the task being practiced. For example, accelerometers on the arm may trigger stimulation to elbow and finger extensors to produce reaching and hand opening when a patient makes an attempt to reach forward (eg, flex the shoulder).[42]

Novel strategies provide users control of not only the timing of stimulation but also the intensity of stimulation, to create an even stronger sense of restored motor control. One such method is called contralaterally controlled functional electrical stimulation (CCFES).[43] With CCFES, a glove with bend sensors is worn on the unaffected hand of a patient with upper extremity hemiparesis. The sensorized glove controls the intensity of stimulation delivered to the finger and thumb extensors of the paretic hand. In this way, a stroke patient has control of the degree of stimulation to the affected hand, allowing varying the amount of hand opening required for any given task that is practiced. In a study comparing CCFES and cyclic NMES in patients with chronic upper limb hemiplegia, 12 weeks of CCFES therapy was shown to improve gross manual dexterity more than the same dose of cyclic NMES therapy.[44]

A recent review of 31 randomized controlled trials (RCTs) concluded that there is strong evidence that NMES applied in the context of task practice improves volitional upper extremity function in subacute and chronic stroke.[45] This is corroborated by a recent meta-analysis of 18 RCTs (9 were upper limb studies) that concluded that NMES-assisted task training has a large therapeutic effect on upper limb activity compared with training alone.[46] The most recent guidelines published by the American Heart Association recommend NMES in combination with task-specific training for stroke rehabilitation.[47]

Neuromodulation for Lower Limb Impairment

Lower limb hemiparesis is one of the most common poststroke impairments.[48] Six months after suffering a stroke, approximately 40% of all stroke survivors are still either unable to walk or require personal assistance to walk even short distances.[49] A major contributor to impaired ambulation is the inability to generate adequate toe clearance during the swing phase of gait, causing the foot to drag, resulting in unsafe and inefficient walking or preventing walking altogether. One of the original applications of NMES was to stimulate the peroneal nerve to dorsiflex the ankle during swing to improve toe clearance in stroke patients.[50]

Three FDA-cleared surface peroneal nerve stimulation (PNS) systems are commercially available: the Odstock Dropped Foot Stimulator (ODFS) (Odstock Medical, Salisbury, United Kingdom), the WalkAide (Innovative Neurotronics, Reno, Nevada), and the NESS L300 (Bioness, Valencia, California). Each device uses surface electrodes, with the active electrode placed over the common peroneal nerve just below the head of the fibula and the return electrode placed over tibialis anterior. A cuff wraps around the upper portion of the shank and contains the surface electrodes and stimulator. A sensor detects the start of swing on the impaired side to trigger stimulation and generate ankle dorsiflexion. The ODFS and NESS L300 both use a wireless heel switch on the paretic side to trigger stimulation when the heel lifts off the ground (ie, at heel-off in the gait cycle). The WalkAide (**Fig. 6**) can be configured to detect step initiation via a heel switch or a tilt sensor built into the cuff to detect forward tilt of the shank resulting from a step with the contralateral limb.

Four large RCTs evaluated the therapeutic and neuroprosthetic effects of surface PNS in comparison to an ankle-foot orthosis (AFO). Three studies evaluated participants after the subacute phase[51–53] and another study focused on patients less than a year poststroke.[54] These studies demonstrated noninferiority, but PNS was not superior to an AFO. When asked about device preference, participants preferred PNS to an AFO because they felt more confident, safer, and more comfortable and found PNS easier to don and doff. Using surface PNS therapeutically for 6 weeks to 30 weeks can significantly improve functional mobility and walking speed. PNS as an assistive device (neuroprosthetic effect) can further improve walking speed and endurance beyond the therapeutic effect. Meta-analyses have shown, however, that PNS devices are neither superior nor inferior to AFOs as orthotic interventions or as therapeutic tools with respect to these outcomes, although some patients may prefer PNS to an AFO.[55,56]

Multijoint Neuromuscular Electrical Stimulation for Hemiparetic Gait

Multichannel systems to assist stroke survivors with greater deficits, such as difficulty flexing and extending the hip and knee, are being developed. The L300 Go (Bioness) has 2 channels of stimulation, which include a PNS cuff and another cuff wrapped around the thigh with electrodes that can be configured to assist either knee flexion or extension (**Fig. 7**). This may be useful if a person cannot generate sufficient knee flexion for toe clearance during swing phase, to assist knee extension for loading and stance, or to reduce hyperextension during stance. Gait events are detected via accelerometers and gyroscopes in the cuffs. The effects of multijoint stimulation were tested in studies using a previous iteration of the device, the L300 Plus (Bioness). A study of 45 participants showed significant therapeutic and neuroprosthetic improvements in walking speed. The addition of knee stimulation to PNS had a statistically significant, but not clinically relevant, additive neuroprosthetic effect on gait speed.[57] Studies evaluating the effect of hamstrings stimulation on kinematics demonstrated a reduction in stance phase hyperextension[58,59] and improved peak swing knee flexion.[59] The participants with less neurologic impairment and spasticity had the greatest response, suggesting greater ability to adapt their volitional movement in response to stimulation.

Patients with greater impairments, such as limited hip range of motion, insufficient knee flexion during swing, inadequate knee extension during stance, or limited push off, may benefit from stimulation of muscles to affect additional joints. An implanted multijoint stimulation system may provide ambulation assistance on a daily basis, in a consistent manner, and with relative ease of use. A case study demonstrated initial feasibility of an implanted neuroprosthesis to improve poststroke gait.[60] A stimulation system incorporating an implantable pulse generator with 8 channels of stimulation connecting to intramuscular electrodes was implanted in hip, knee, and ankle muscles

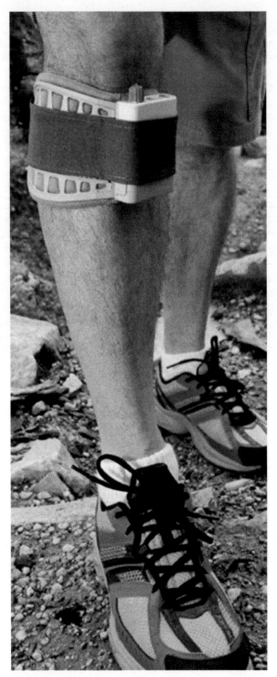

Fig. 6. Walk-aide PNS system for ankle dorsiflexion. (*Courtesy of* Innovative Neurotronics Inc, Reno, NV; with permission.)

(**Fig. 8**). An external controller provided power and commands. A heel switch triggered temporal sequences for swing phase and stance phase stimulation, which were initiated at heel off and heel strike, respectively. Therapeutic improvements in gait speed and spatiotemporal characteristics were statistically significant but modest. Walking

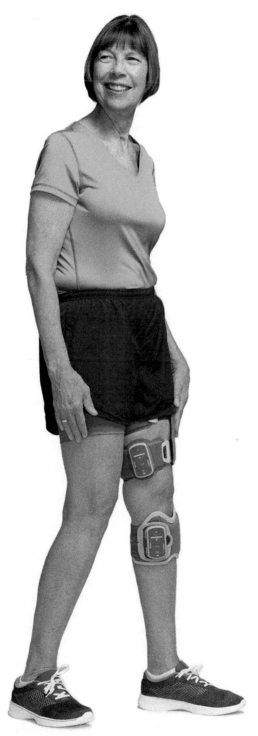

Fig. 7. L300 Go combining surface stimulation for ankle dorsiflexion and knee flexion or extension. (*Courtesy of* Bioness, Inc, Valencia, CA; with permission.)

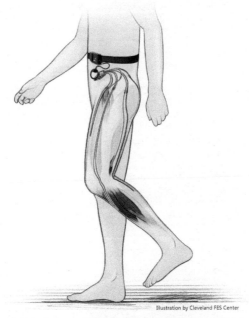

Illustration by Cleveland FES Center

Fig. 8. Implanted and external components of an 8-channel multijoint stimulation system. (*Courtesy of* Cleveland FES Center, Cleveland, OH; with permission.)

with stimulation assistance (ie, the neuroprosthetic effect), however, provided a clinically relevant increase in gait speed (>0.2 m/s) with associated improvements in spatiotemporal characteristics.

SUMMARY

Neuromodulation with electrical stimulation has allowed significant improvements in function for those who have experienced disability due to SCI and stroke. There are many clinical problems that still require treatments. Future directions will focus on improving existing technology to give the user an experience closer to neurointact function, including closed-loop systems in which physiologic monitoring can alter the neuromodulatory effects of electrical stimulation without user intervention. Other technologies under development are restoration of sensation, reduction in spasticity and pain, and improvement of organ function. Aside from technological advancement, innovations in bringing these devices to the disabled population are needed. Such innovations could include nonprofit support of device development for orphan populations or finding indications for novel treatments to expand the market to reduce costs. Despite the challenges, neuromodulation will remain one of the best options to reduce disabilities related to neurologic injury or illness.

REFERENCES

1. Anderson KD. Targeting recovery: priorities of the spinal cord-injured population. J Neurotrauma 2004;21(10):1371–83.
2. Creasey GH, Grill JH, Korsten M, et al. An implantable neuroprosthesis for restoring bladder and bowel control to patients with spinal cord injuries: a multi-center trial. Arch Phys Med Rehabil 2001;82(11):1512–9.

3. Onders RP, Elmo M, Khansarinia S, et al. Complete worldwide operative experience in laparoscopic diaphragm pacing: results and differences in spinal cord injured patients and amyotrophic lateral sclerosis patients. Surg Endosc 2009; 23(7):1433–40.

4. DiMarco AF, Onders RP, Ignagni A, et al. Phrenic nerve pacing via intramuscular diaphragm electrodes in tetraplegic subjects. Chest 2005;127(2):671–8.

5. DiMarco AF, Kowalski KE, Geertman RT, et al. Lower thoracic spinal cord stimulation to restore cough in patients with spinal cord injury: results of a national institutes of health-sponsored clinical trial. Part I: methodology and effectiveness of expiratory muscle activation. Arch Phys Med Rehabil 2009;90(5):717–25.

6. Kilgore KL, Hoyen HA, Bryden AM, et al. An implanted upper-extremity neuroprosthesis using myoelectric control. J Hand Surg 2008;33(4):539–50.

7. Peckham PH, Keith MW, Kilgore KL, et al. Efficacy of an implanted neuroprosthesis for restoring hand grasp in tetraplegia: a multicenter study. Arch Phys Med Rehabil 2001;82(10):1380–8.

8. Bryden AM, Memberg WD, Crago PE. Electrically stimulated elbow extension in persons with C5/C6 tetraplegia: a functional and physiological evaluation. Arch Phys Med Rehabil 2000;81(1):80–8.

9. Triolo RJ, Bailey SN, Lombardo LM, et al. Effects of intramuscular trunk stimulation on manual wheelchair propulsion mechanics in 6 subjects with spinal cord injury. Arch Phys Med Rehabil 2013;94(10):1997–2005.

10. Triolo RJ, Boggs L, Miller ME, et al. Implanted electrical stimulation of the trunk for seated postural stability and function after cervical spinal cord injury: a single case study. Arch Phys Med Rehabil 2009;90(2):340–7.

11. Triolo RJ, Bailey SN, Miller ME, et al. Longitudinal performance of a surgically implanted neuroprosthesis for lower-extremity exercise, standing, and transfers after spinal cord injury. Arch Phys Med Rehabil 2012;93(5):896–904.

12. Lombardo LM, Bailey SN, Foglyano KM, et al. A preliminary comparison of myoelectric and cyclic control of an implanted neuroprosthesis to modulate gait speed in incomplete. J Spinal Cord Med 2015;38(1):115–22.

13. Triolo RJ, Bailey SN, Foglyano KM, et al. Long-term performance and user satisfaction with implanted neuroprostheses for upright mobility after paraplegia: 2- to 14-year follow-up. Arch Phys Med Rehabil 2018;99(2):289–98.

14. Peckham PH, Kilgore KL. Challenges and opportunities in restoring function after paralysis. IEEE Trans Biomed Eng 2013;60(3):602–9.

15. Middleton JW, Lim K, Taylor L, et al. Patterns of morbidity and rehospitalisation following spinal cord injury. Spinal Cord 2004;42(6):359–67.

16. Siegel SW, Catanzaro F, Dijkema HE, et al. Long-term results of a multicenter study on sacral nerve stimulation for treatment of urinary urge incontinence, urgency-frequency, and retention. Urology 2000;56(6 Suppl 1):87–91.

17. Govier FE, Litwiller S, Nitti V, et al. Percutaneous afferent neuromodulation for the refractory overactive bladder: results of a multicenter study. J Urol 2001;165(4): 1193–8.

18. Sievert K-D, Amend B, Gakis G, et al. Early sacral neuromodulation prevents urinary incontinence after complete spinal cord injury. Ann Neurol 2010;67(1): 74–84.

19. Bourbeau DJ, Creasey GH, Sidik S, et al. Genital nerve stimulation increases bladder capacity after SCI: a meta-analysis. J Spinal Cord Med 2018;41(4): 426–34.

20. Opisso E, Borau A, Rijkhoff NJM. Subject-controlled stimulation of dorsal genital nerve to treat neurogenic detrusor overactivity at home. Neurourol Urodyn 2013; 32(7):1004–9.
21. Bourbeau DJ, Gustafson KJ, Brose SW. At-home genital nerve stimulation for individuals with SCI and neurogenic detrusor overactivity: a pilot feasibility study. J Spinal Cord Med 2018;1–11. https://doi.org/10.1080/10790268.2017.1422881.
22. Creasey GH. Electrical stimulation of sacral roots for micturition after spinal cord injury. Urol Clin North Am 1993;20(3):505–15.
23. Boger AS, Bhadra N, Gustafson KJ. High frequency sacral root nerve block allows bladder voiding. Neurourol Urodyn 2012;31(5):677–82.
24. Carter RE, Donovan WH, Halstead L, et al. Comparative study of electrophrenic nerve stimulation and mechanical ventilatory support in traumatic spinal cord injury. Paraplegia 1987;25(2):86–91.
25. DiMarco AF. Diaphragm pacing. Clin Chest Med 2018;39(2):459–71.
26. Lam JC, Ho CT, Poon TL, et al. Implantation of a breathing pacemaker in a tetraplegic patient in Hong Kong. Hong Kong Med J 2009;15(3):230–3.
27. Krieger LM, Krieger AJ. The intercostal to phrenic nerve transfer: an effective means of reanimating the diaphragm in patients with high cervical spine injury. Plast Reconstr Surg 2000;105(4):1255–61.
28. Elefteriades JA, Quin JA, Hogan JF, et al. Long-term follow-up of pacing of the conditioned diaphragm in quadriplegia. Pacing Clin Electrophysiol 2002;25(6): 897–906.
29. Glenn WW, Phelps ML, Elefteriades JA, et al. Twenty years of experience in phrenic nerve stimulation to pace the diaphragm. Pacing Clin Electrophysiol 1986;9(6 Pt 1):780–4.
30. DiMarco AF, Kowalski KE. Activation of inspiratory muscles via spinal cord stimulation. Respir Physiol Neurobiol 2013;189(2):438–49.
31. Bach JR, Saporito LR, Shah HR, et al. Decanulation of patients with severe respiratory muscle insufficiency: efficacy of mechanical insufflation-exsufflation. J Rehabil Med 2014;46(10):1037–41.
32. DiMarco AF. Restoration of respiratory muscle function following spinal cord injury. Review of electrical and magnetic stimulation techniques. Respir Physiol Neurobiol 2005;147(2–3):273–87.
33. Butler JE, Lim J, Gorman RB, et al. Posterolateral surface electrical stimulation of abdominal expiratory muscles to enhance cough in spinal cord injury. Neurorehabil Neural Repair 2011;25(2):158–67.
34. DiMarco AF, Geertman RT, Tabbaa K, et al. Economic consequences of an implanted neuroprosthesis in subjects with spinal cord injury for restoration of an effective cough. Top Spinal Cord Inj Rehabil 2017;23(3):271–8.
35. Teasell R, Bitensky J, Salter K, et al. The role of timing and intensity of rehabilitation therapies. Top Stroke Rehabil 2005;12(3):46–57.
36. Hsu SS, Hu MH, Luh JJ, et al. Dosage of neuromuscular electrical stimulation: is it a determinant of upper limb functional improvement in stroke patients? J Rehabil Med 2012;44(2):125–30.
37. Rosewilliam S, Malhotra S, Roffe C, et al. Can surface neuromuscular electrical stimulation of the wrist and hand combined with routine therapy facilitate recovery of arm function in patients with stroke? Arch Phys Med Rehabil 2012;93(10): 1715–21.e1.
38. Alon G, Levitt AF, McCarthy PA. Functional electrical stimulation enhancement of upper extremity functional recovery during stroke rehabilitation: a pilot study. Neurorehabil Neural Repair 2007;21(3):207–15.

39. Thrasher TA, Zivanovic V, McIlroy W, et al. Rehabilitation of reaching and grasping function in severe hemiplegic patients using functional electrical stimulation therapy. Neurorehabil Neural Repair 2008;22(6):706–14.

40. Meilink A, Hemmen B, Seelen HA, et al. Impact of EMG-triggered neuromuscular stimulation of the wrist and finger extensors of the paretic hand after stroke: a systematic review of the literature. Clin Rehabil 2008;22(4):291–305.

41. Rushton DN. Functional electrical stimulation and rehabilitation–an hypothesis. Med Eng Phys 2003;25(1):75–8.

42. Mann G, Taylor P, Lane R. Accelerometer-triggered electrical stimulation for reach and grasp in chronic stroke patients: a pilot study. Neurorehabil Neural Repair 2011;25(8):774–80.

43. Knutson JS, Harley MY, Hisel TZ, et al. Improving hand function in stroke survivors: a pilot study of contralaterally controlled functional electric stimulation in chronic hemiplegia. Arch Phys Med Rehabil 2007;88(4):513–20.

44. Knutson JS, Gunzler DD, Wilson RD, et al. Contralaterally controlled functional electrical stimulation improves hand dexterity in chronic hemiparesis: a randomized trial. Stroke 2016;47:2596–602.

45. Foley N, Mehta S, Jutai J, et al. Upper extremity interventions. In: Teasell R, editor. Evidence-based review of stroke rehabilitation. 16th edition. London: Heart & Stroke Foundation Canadian Partnership for Stroke Recovery; 2014. p. 1–208.

46. Howlett OA, Lannin NA, Ada L, et al. Functional electrical stimulation improves activity after stroke: a systematic review with meta-analysis. Arch Phys Med Rehabil 2015;96(5):934–43.

47. Winstein CJ, Stein J, Arena R, et al. Guidelines for adult stroke rehabilitation and recovery: a guideline for healthcare professionals from the American Heart Association/American Stroke Association. Stroke 2016;47(6):e98–169.

48. Lai SM, Studenski S, Duncan PW, et al. Persisting consequences of stroke measured by the Stroke Impact Scale. Stroke 2002;33(7):1840–4.

49. Jorgensen HS, Nakayama H, Raaschou HO, et al. Recovery of walking function in stroke patients: the Copenhagen Stroke Study. Arch Phys Med Rehabil 1995; 76(1):27–32.

50. Liberson WT, Holmquest HJ, Scot D, et al. Functional electrotherapy: stimulation of the peroneal nerve synchronized with the swing phase of the gait of hemiplegic patients. Arch Phys Med Rehabil 1961;42:101–5.

51. Sheffler LR, Taylor PN, Gunzler DD, et al. Randomized controlled trial of surface peroneal nerve stimulation for motor relearning in lower limb hemiparesis. Arch Phys Med Rehabil 2013;94(6):1007–14.

52. Kluding PM, Dunning K, O'Dell MW, et al. Foot drop stimulation versus ankle foot orthosis after stroke: 30-week outcomes. Stroke 2013;44(6):1660–9.

53. Bethoux F, Rogers HL, Nolan KJ, et al. The effects of peroneal nerve functional electrical stimulation versus ankle-foot orthosis in patients with chronic stroke: a randomized controlled trial. Neurorehabil Neural Repair 2014;28(7):688–97.

54. Everaert DG, Stein RB, Abrams GM, et al. Effect of a foot-drop stimulator and ankle-foot orthosis on walking performance after stroke: a multicenter randomized controlled trial. Neurorehabil Neural Repair 2013;27(7):579–91.

55. Prenton S, Hollands KL, Kenney LPJ, et al. Functional electrical stimulation and ankle foot orthoses provide equivalent therapeutic effects on foot drop: a meta-analysis providing direction for future research. J Rehabil Med 2018;50(2): 129–39.

56. Prenton S, Hollands KL, Kenney LP. Functional electrical stimulation versus ankle foot orthoses for foot-drop: a meta-analysis of orthotic effects. J Rehabil Med 2016;48(8):646–56.

57. Springer S, Vatine JJ, Lipson R, et al. Effects of dual-channel functional electrical stimulation on gait performance in patients with hemiparesis. ScientificWorldJournal 2012;2012:530906.

58. Springer S, Vatine JJ, Wolf A, et al. The effects of dual-channel functional electrical stimulation on stance phase sagittal kinematics in patients with hemiparesis. J Electromyogr Kinesiol 2013;23(2):476–82.

59. Tenniglo MJ, Buurke JH, Prinsen EC, et al. Influence of functional electrical stimulation of the hamstrings on knee kinematics in stroke survivors walking with stiff knee gait. J Rehabil Med 2018;50(8):719–24.

60. Makowski NS, Kobetic R, Lombardo LM, et al. Improving walking with an implanted neuroprosthesis for hip, knee, and ankle control after stroke. Am J Phys Med Rehabil 2016;95(12):880–8.

Noninvasive Transcranial Magnetic Brain Stimulation in Stroke

Julio C. Hernandez-Pavon, PhD, DSc[a,b], Richard L. Harvey, MD[a,c],*

KEYWORDS

• Noninvasive • Transcranial magnetic stimulation • Stroke • Rehabilitation

KEY POINTS

• It is likely that transcranial magnetic brain stimulation will be used for the clinical treatment of stroke and stroke-related impairments in the future.
• The anatomic target and stimulation parameters will likely vary for any clinical focus, be it weakness, pain, or cognitive or communicative dysfunction.
• Biomarkers may also be useful for identifying patients who will respond best, with a goal to enhance clinical decision making.
• Combination with drugs or specific types of therapeutic exercise may be necessary to achieve maximal response.

INTRODUCTION

Modern approaches to therapeutic exercise in stroke rehabilitation can accelerate the recovery of motor control and function but still do not typically lead to complete recovery in patients with moderate to severe stroke.[1,2] As a result, clinical neuroscientists have turned to technology coupled with therapeutic task practice to facilitate further neural recovery.[3] This article discusses the emerging use of neuromodulation in the form of noninvasive electromagnetic brain stimulation. Transcranial magnetic stimulation (TMS) presently has few clinical applications. However, TMS could potentially have wide use in stroke rehabilitation if clinicians can identify effective stimulation parameters. As shown in this review, there are several different therapeutic stimulation parameters under investigation, and each may ultimately have a clinical role depending on the neurologic condition.

Disclosure: The authors have nothing to disclose.
[a] Department of Physical Medicine and Rehabilitation, Feinberg School of Medicine, Northwestern University, Chicago, IL, USA; [b] Center for Brain Stimulation, Shirley Ryan AbilityLab, 355 East Erie Street, Chicago, IL 60611, USA; [c] Brain Innovation Center, Shirley Ryan AbilityLab, 355 East Erie Street, Chicago, IL 60611, USA
* Corresponding author. Shirley Ryan Abilitylab, 355 East Erie Street, Chicago, IL 60611, USA.
E-mail address: rharvey@sralab.org

Phys Med Rehabil Clin N Am 30 (2019) 319–335
https://doi.org/10.1016/j.pmr.2018.12.010
1047-9651/19/© 2019 Elsevier Inc. All rights reserved.

BASIC PRINCIPLES OF TRANSCRANIAL MAGNETIC STIMULATION

TMS is a powerful technique to noninvasively stimulate the human brain.[4] In TMS, a strong and time-varying magnetic pulse is delivered to the brain by means of a coil.[5] These coils consist of a small number of turns of copper wire tightly wound in an insulating material. The magnetic pulse produced by the coil induces an electric field in the cortex and this produces neuronal activation when pyramidal cells and inhibitory interneurons are depolarized.[6,7] The physical principle of TMS is based on electromagnetic induction, described by Faraday's law, whereby a changing magnetic field (**B**) induces an electric field (**E**). If the magnetic field changes slowly or is static, no neuronal excitation occurs. The strength of the magnetic field used in TMS is on the order of 1 to 2 T and its rise time is approximately 100 microseconds.

The magnetic pulse in TMS is generated by passing a current pulse through an induction coil placed over the scalp. The basic circuit of the magnetic stimulator is simple and consists of a capacitor (C) connected in series with the stimulation coil (inductor L) by a thyristor (switch). Because there is resistance (R) in the coil, cables, thyristor, and capacitor, the circuit forms an RLC oscillator system. The capacitor is first charged to between 2 and 3 kV and then discharged by the gating of the thyristor, producing a current pulse with a peak value of 5 to 10 kA.[6] At present, more sophisticated stimulators and multichannel TMS systems are under development for stimulating multiple brain areas.[8]

TMS activates neurons in the cortex rather than deeper parts of the brain. In addition to the target area, TMS activates distant interconnected sites in the brain, which has been shown to be important for studies of brain connectivity.[5] The temporal resolution of TMS is submilliseconds, which allows for real-time modulation of the brain. The spatial distribution of the induced electric field in the brain varies from several millimeters up to centimeters and it depends on the shape and the location of the coil. In addition, the orientation of the coil with respect to the tissue and the electrical conductivity of the tissue contribute to the size of the electric field.[6,9] Most of the TMS coils are not designed to stimulate deep brain areas and only are able to stimulate cortical areas under the wing junction (figure-of-eight coil) or under the windings of the coil (circular coil).[6] Nevertheless, the double-cone coil[10] and Hesed or H coil[11] have been shown to be effective in reaching between 3 and 4 cm in depth, allowing stimulation of deeper brain areas such as the leg motor area. The double-cone coil is a modified version of the figure-of-eight coil in which the angle between the 2 wings is approximately 95° to 120°, whereas the H coil is a more sophisticated design whereby the main characteristic is to stimulate deeper brain regions without increasing the electric field intensity in the cortical areas.[10–12]

At the microscopic level, TMS forces free charges in intracellular and extracellular volumes to move by the electric field. The magnetic field has no direct effect on ions; the effect is produced by the electric field, which affects the drift on ions and orients dipoles. The chain of events in TMS is depicted in **Fig. 1**. The stimulation produced by TMS opens up unique possibilities to map the human brain, which can be done at the system level on sensory, cognitive, and motor brain networks. Therefore, combining TMS with various neuroimaging techniques, such as electroencephalography (EEG),[5,13] functional MRI,[14] PET,[15] or near-infrared spectroscopy,[16] allows clinicians to investigate human brain functions.

MRI-guided navigated TMS (nTMS) has become the state of the art in performing TMS studies because the stimulation is more accurate and reproducible.[17,18] The use of coil trackers and a subject-worn head tracker system enables the recording of the relative position between the head of the subject and the TMS coil in real

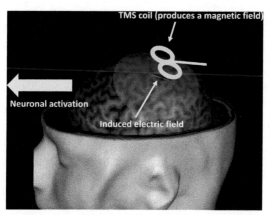

Fig. 1. Chain of events caused by TMS. A strong magnetic pulse is generated by the flow of electric currents in the TMS coil. The magnetic field induces an electric field in the brain (the red and blue arrows show the direction of the induced electric field). The electric field produces the movement of ions in the membrane of the pyramidal axons, leading to depolarization and subsequent neuronal activation.

time.[18] With nTMS, the individual's brain MRI allows the stimulated cortical target to be accurately defined anatomically. In addition, the coil position can be monitored, and the orientation and, in some systems, the strength of the induced electric field can also be estimated in real time. These factors are important features that contribute to reproducibility.[19,20]

PHYSIOLOGIC EFFECT OF SINGLE-PULSE AND REPETITIVE TRANSCRANIAL MAGNETIC STIMULATION
Single-Pulse Transcranial Magnetic Stimulation

When stimuli are applied at a low rate so that the activity produced by previous pulses does not interfere with that of the new pulse, the stimulation is considered single-pulse TMS; the rate of these pulses is lower than 1 Hz.

Most knowledge about the effects of single-pulse TMS on the human cortex comes from studies performed on the primary motor cortex (M1).[21] Stimulation of M1 evokes activity in muscles on the opposite side of the body, which can be measured by using electromyography (EMG).[4] In contrast, stimulation of most other parts of the cortex (at least with single pulses) has no obvious effects. One exception is the stimulation of the visual cortex, which can elicit phosphenes.[22,23]

TMS of M1 exhibits 2 effects that are likely to also occur when stimulating other cortical areas. The size of the response depends on the level of activity in the cortex at the time the stimulus is given, and it depends on the orientation of the TMS coil.[7] The orientation of the coil plays an important role in the response because pyramidal neurons are oriented mainly perpendicular to the cortical surface.[24,25] Depending on the folding of the cortex, the neurons have specific orientations with respect to the TMS-induced currents that favor one or another population of neurons.[26–28] As a consequence of this, the activation of the hand area of the motor cortex occurs at the lowest threshold when the stimulus induces posterior to anterior currents perpendicular to the central sulcus.[29]

At the neuronal level, when a single TMS pulse is delivered to the motor cortex, it induces a firing activity in the intracortical interneurons. This activity has been directly recorded by epidural electrodes placed over the cervical spinal cord, suggesting that this activity or series of volleys are separated from each other by about

1.5 milliseconds (~670 Hz).[21,30] The initial volley is called D wave (direct wave) and is generated by direct stimulation of the axons of the large pyramidal track neurons in layer V (**Fig. 2**). The later volleys are the I waves (indirect waves), which originate from indirect activation of the large pyramidal track neurons through trans-synaptic activation of layers II and III (see **Fig. 2**).[21,30] Different combinations of D and I waves can be induced depending on the coil orientation, pulse waveform, stimulation intensity, and the level of voluntary muscle contraction.[21,30]

Repetitive Transcranial Magnetic Stimulation

When a train of pulses is delivered, the TMS technique is called repetitive TMS (rTMS). Low-frequency rTMS refers to a train of pulses at frequencies of less than or equal to 1 Hz that tends to have an inhibitory effect,[31] whereas high-frequency rTMS refers to a train of pulses delivered at frequencies greater than 5 Hz and that have typically been found to have an excitatory effect[32–34] (**Fig. 3**).

rTMS can induce persistent effects on the brain. The duration of the after-effects is often 30 to 60 minutes but depends on properties such as the number of pulses applied, the frequency or stimulation rate, and the intensity of each stimulus. Because of the effects of rTMS that outlast the stimulation, this technique has generated a lot of interest as a method to study cognitive processes and as a potential therapeutic tool for the treatment of neurologic and psychiatric disorders.[35]

The physiologic bases of rTMS after-effects remain unclear. However, evidence from animal studies suggests that the mechanisms underlying rTMS after-effects might be associated with long-term potentiation and long-term depression. In addition, the effects of rTMS in increasing or decreasing motor cortical excitability have recently been investigated by recording responses of the corticospinal volley evoked by single-pulse TMS before and after different rTMS protocols.[36]

Repetitive Transcranial Magnetic Stimulation Safety

Although rTMS is generally safe, there is a risk of seizures when rTMS is applied at coil intensities greater than the motor threshold, high frequencies, and short interval

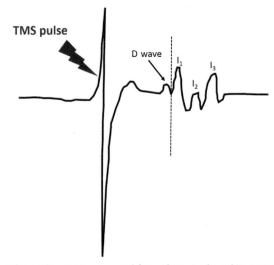

Fig. 2. TMS-induced D and I waves measured from the spinal cord in response to a TMS pulse delivered over the motor cortex. The D and I waves lead to the motor evoked responses.

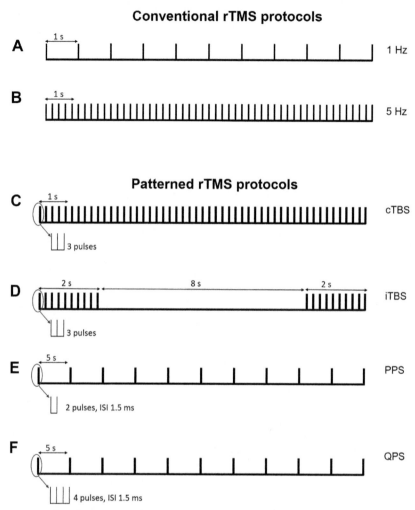

Fig. 3. Examples of conventional and patterned rTMS protocols. Conventional rTMS protocols consist of identical stimuli spaced by an identical interstimulus interval (ISI) between the delivered pulses. Patterned rTMS protocols are characterized by different ISIs within a train of pulses. For example, theta-burst stimulation (TBS) consists of pulses applied in bursts of 3 at 50 Hz with an interburst interval at 5 Hz. In paired-pulse stimulation, a burst of 2 pulses is delivered with a 1.5-millisecond ISI with an interburst interval of 0.2 Hz (or 5 seconds). Quadropulse stimulation delivers 4 pulses with a 1.5-millisecond ISI and a 0.2-Hz interburst interval. Of note, in PPS and QPS, the length of ISI can be varied. (*A*) Low-frequency rTMS (1 Hz); (*B*) high-frequency rTMS (5 Hz); (*C*) continuous TBS (cTBS); (*D*) intermittent TBS (iTBS; 2 seconds of TBS are delivered every 10 seconds); (*E*) paired-pulse stimulation (PPS); (*F*) quadropulse stimulation (QPS).

periods between trains of stimulation exceeding the known safety limits reported in the literature.[37,38] From the first use of rTMS until 2008, a total of 16 seizures were reported.[38] A recent review published in 2015 identified 25 incidences of seizures,[39] of which 19 cases were caused by high-frequency rTMS, 4 cases by multiple single-pulse stimulations, 1 with continuous theta-burst stimulation (TBS), and 1 not reported.[39] Despite the number of seizures reported so far, the reported risk of seizures remains at 1 in 1000 applications. The main factors that seem to induced rTMS seizures are high-frequency rTMS, motor cortex stimulation, preexisting conditions, sleep deprivation, polypharmacy, and previous seizure history.[38,39] Therefore, caution is needed while using rTMS and the rTMS guidelines should be followed.[37,38]

The only absolute contraindication to TMS/rTMS is the presence of metallic hardware anywhere in the head (excluding the mouth) or anywhere in the body in close contact with the TMS coil (eg, cochlear implants, neurostimulators, pacemakers, or medical pumps).[38]

In addition, there are several conditions that might increase the risk of inducing epileptic seizures and therefore are part of the exclusion criteria of patients and healthy participants (eg, personal history of epilepsy; vascular, traumatic, neoplastic, infectious, or metabolic lesions of the brain; sleep deprivation; alcoholism; drugs that potentially increase excitability). Other conditions of increased or uncertain risk include implanted brain electrodes (either cortical or deep-brain electrodes), pregnancy, severe or recent heart disease, recent brain surgery, and history of serious head trauma.[38]

REPETITIVE TRANSCRANIAL MAGNETIC STIMULATION PROTOCOLS IN STROKE

The aim here is not to extensively review all the clinical studies published in the literature. Instead, the goal is to provide a general overview of the parameters used in the different rTMS protocols for treating stroke, in particular for upper limb recovery. The use of rTMS following a stroke is based on the interhemispheric inhibition model, whereby excitability in the affected hemisphere is reduced and excitability in the unaffected hemisphere is increased.[40,41] After a stroke, the activity in the affected hemisphere is also disrupted by an increase in the transcallosal inhibition from the unaffected hemisphere, which further reduces the excitability of the affected hemisphere.

Because of the ability of rTMS to neuromodulate the human brain by either increasing or decreasing cortical excitability, the rTMS protocols used in stroke can be divided into 2 groups. Excitatory or facilitatory protocols are those in which rTMS is used to increase the cortical excitability of the affected hemisphere, whereas inhibitory protocols are those in which rTMS aims to reduce the excitability of the unaffected hemisphere.[40] The main hypothesis is that low-frequency or inhibitory rTMS over the unaffected hemisphere reduces transcallosal inhibition from the unaffected hemisphere to the affected hemisphere, and high-frequency or facilitatory rTMS over the affected hemisphere increases transcallosal inhibition from the affected to the unaffected hemisphere.[42]

Excitatory Protocols

High-frequency repetitive transcranial magnetic stimulation
Following the interhemispheric inhibition model, high-frequency rTMS has been delivered to the affected hemisphere to increase cortical excitability and, therefore, to improve motor functions following a stroke.[43] rTMS has been applied at frequencies of 3, 10, or 20 Hz in single or multiple sessions at different intensities from 80% to 130% resting motor threshold.[43,44]

Intermittent theta-burst stimulation
A modified form of rTMS is TBS, which consists of pulses applied in bursts of 3 at 50 Hz with an interburst interval at 5 Hz.[45,46] When 2 seconds of TBS are delivered every 10 seconds, this technique is called intermittent TBS (iTBS) and has excitatory effects[45,46] (see **Fig. 3**). The main advantages of iTBS compared with high-frequency

rTMS are the lower stimulus intensities required and the shorter application times. Therefore, iTBS seems to be a promising tool for increasing excitability of the unaffected hemisphere of patients with stroke. In addition, iTBS is less likely to induce seizure compared with high-frequency rTMS, in which long periods of stimulation and high stimulation intensities are required. In healthy participants, iTBS has been shown to be effective in increasing cortical excitability for 20 minutes.[45] iTBS parameters in stroke are 20 trains of 10 bursts (600 pulses) with intertrain intervals of 8 or 10 seconds at 80% of the active motor threshold (AMT).[43]

Inhibitory Protocols

Low-frequency repetitive transcranial magnetic stimulation

Low-frequency rTMS over the unaffected hemisphere has been widely used to suppress cortical excitability and consequently reduce transcallosal inhibition to the affected hemisphere.[47] In a typical low-frequency rTMS protocol, 600 to 1800 rTMS pulses are delivered at stimulation intensities from 90% to 120% resting motor threshold in single or multiple sessions.[48] The effect of delivering up to 2400 rTMS pulses has recently been investigated.[49]

Continuous theta-burst stimulation

Continuous TBS (cTBS) administered to the unaffected hemisphere is another inhibitory protocol used in stroke (see **Fig. 3**). In cTBS, uninterrupted TBS pulses are delivered for 20 or 40 seconds.[45,46] The stimulation intensities used in cTBS protocols are 70% to 80% AMT and the number of pulses varies from 150 to 600.[50]

Paired-Pulse and Quadropulse Transcranial Magnetic Stimulation

Repetitive paired-pulse TMS (PPS) is the other promising rTMS protocol for neuromodulation. In PPS, paired TMS pulses of equal intensity with an interstimulus interval (ISI) of 1.5 milliseconds are delivered at 0.2 Hz (every 5 seconds[51] see **Fig. 3**). In healthy participants, 30 minutes of PPS increased the amplitude of motor evoked potentials (MEPs) up to 10 minutes after the stimulation.[51] New evidence suggests that the ISI and frequency might play a role in increasing or decreasing cortical excitability.[52] However, its application has been limited for treating stroke and there are not enough data on the outcome.

Quadropulse stimulation (QPS) is a modification of the PPS protocol.[53] In QPS, 4 pulses are delivered with an ISI of 1.5 milliseconds at 0.2 Hz[52,53] (see **Fig. 3**). In healthy participants, 30 minutes of QPS reduced the amplitude of the MEP for about 75 minutes.[52,53] Despite the possible potential of QPS to neuromodulate cortical excitability, its application has also been limited in stroke by variability in responses of the motor cortex.[54]

CLINICAL USES OF REPETITIVE TRANSCRANIAL MAGNETIC STIMULATION IN STROKE

High-frequency rTMS was approved for the treatment of drug-resistant depression in the United States in 2008 following a 2007 randomized sham-controlled pivotal trial, and its effectiveness has been supported by a more recent meta-analysis of trials using both high and low frequency protocols.[55,56] Furthermore, rTMS can be used to treat poststroke depression in patients who fail to respond to drug treatment.[57] There is evidence that suggests that rTMS may have many other clinical uses for the treatment of stroke. This article now briefly reviews the current evidence for treatment of other stroke-related impairments, including hemiplegia, dysphagia, neglect syndrome, and central poststroke pain.

Hemiplegia

A most challenging problem in stroke rehabilitation is restoration of arm and hand function. Only 20% of patients recover normal hand function and less than 50% use the affected arm and hand in any activity.[58] Although most patients walk after stroke, only 50% recover independent community ambulation.[59]

The conceptual framework for the use of rTMS in the treatment of hemiplegia is to reduce interhemispheric inhibition, whereby an injury to cerebral hemisphere causes not only a low level of cortical excitability in perilesional surviving cortex but leads to a hyperexcitable contralateral motor cortex. Balance can be restored either by direct upregulation of surviving perilesional cortex or by downregulation of the noninjured hemisphere, which then reduces inhibitory drive.[60] The theoretic impact is the modulation of cortical neuronal activity in order to achieve maximum facilitation of adaptive neuroplastic changes in the perilesional cortex. This theory is justified because the return of balance in cortical excitability between hemispheres is associated with motor recovery poststroke and may be necessary for effective restoration of skilled motor performance.[61,62]

Direct upregulation of an injured hemisphere can be achieved with an ipsilateral excitatory TMS protocol. High-frequency rTMS results in an increase in MEP amplitude and resting motor threshold within the perilesional cortex.[63–65] In laboratory studies, a single session of high-frequency rTMS targeting an arm and hand representation of the ipsilesional cortex can induce transient improvement of finger dexterity and hand grip in patients with chronic stroke.[64,66–68] Khedr and colleagues[69] conducted a randomized clinical trial comparing 300 pulses of 3-Hz rTMS to injured hemisphere with sham therapy in 52 patients with acute stroke, showing better neurologic and functional recovery in treated subjects as measured by the National Institutes of Health Stroke Scale, Scandinavian Stroke Scale, and Barthel Index. Patients who have superior upper limb motor outcomes following a course of high-frequency rTMS tend to have better cortical spinal tract integrity and are positive for the brain-derived neurotrophic factor (BDNF) val66met polymorphism.[70]

The use of inhibitory TMS protocols such as low-frequency rTMS to the noninjured hemisphere might be considered a more attractive alternative for motor rehabilitation in stroke because it is easier to target motor regions in healthy cortex and the risk of inducing seizures is lower. Small, randomized trials have supported the efficacy of 1-Hz rTMS to the noninjured hemisphere, showing improvements in finger tapping, pinch force, and hand acceleration.[71,72] These motor improvements are associated with corticospinal excitability changes in perilesional cortex, suggesting effective reduction of interhemispheric inhibition.[60] A meta-analysis of 22 trials of low-frequency rTMS for poststroke hemiplegia confirms a positive impact on hemiplegic hand dexterity, strength, and flexibility.[48] However, a recent large randomized clinical trial by Harvey and colleagues[73] failed to show any benefit of low-frequency rTMS when combined with a standardized task-oriented hand-skill rehabilitation program. This study included 199 subjects 3 to 12 months poststroke, for which analysis was completed on 173 subjects because of early study termination due to statistical futility. Both treatment groups (1-Hz rTMS targeted to motor cortex vs sham) had significant improvements in upper limb motor control based on change in Fugl-Meyer score from baseline to 6-month follow-up (combined outcome of 8.2 ± 8.1 points) with no between-group differences. This equivocal outcome may have been caused by a strong impact from the rehabilitation therapy versus effective neuromodulation induced by the nontargeted low electric field delivered by the sham coil used in the trial.

There have been only a few trials testing the efficacy of rTMS for restoration of lower limb function and walking skill, from a single laboratory in Korea. These investigators have found that high-frequency rTMS to injured motor cortex combined with therapy can improve gait speed and cadence compared with sham treatment in patients with both acute and chronic stroke.[74–76] Wang and colleagues[77] combined low-frequency rTMS with lower limb exercise and gait training in a randomized trial showing that combined treatment improved gait speed, symmetry, step length, and cadence compared with sham rTMS and training. Others have had promising findings using modified coil designs such as the double-cone coil and the H coil for achieving deep motor cortex stimulation to improve walking.[78,79]

There is some published work on the use of TBS for motor recovery after stroke. Talelli and colleagues[80] showed that excitatory iTBS to injured hemisphere motor cortex could improve hand reaction time in subjects with chronic stroke. In contrast, inhibitory cTBS to noninjured hemisphere did not improve reaction time. In a subsequent randomized clinical trial, this group failed to show any effect of iTBS or cTBS compared with sham when combined with therapy.[81] In another randomized clinical trial, Kondo and colleagues[49] found stimulation to noninjured hemisphere with low-frequency rTMS superior to cTBS for motor recovery when combined with arm and hand rehabilitation.

Three trials have tested the combined use of excitatory and inhibitory TMS protocols, to injured and noninjured hemispheres respectively, and the results support superiority compared with unilateral treatment with repetitive TMS.[82–84] More work evaluating the efficacy of bilateral TMS therapy for hemiplegia is needed.

The most recent Cochrane Review on the use of rTMS for motor recovery dates back to 2013. Hao and colleagues[85] reviewed 19 trials including 588 patients, and found no significant safety concerns. They also found no significant effect of rTMS modalities on motor recovery or improvement in overall function (Barthel Index). In a more recent meta-analysis focusing on rTMS for upper limb recovery, which included 9 studies with 289 patients, Ling and colleagues[86] found supportive evidence that especially low-frequency rTMS was beneficial for recovery of arm and hand and that rTMS is safe to use in patients with stroke.

Dysphagia

Recovery of swallowing after stroke is an important goal for up to 67% of patients who have dysphagia.[87] Hamdy and colleagues[88] have shown that muscles of the pharynx have an asymmetric somatotopic representation in the motor and premotor areas of both hemispheres, suggesting a cortical dominance that is unrelated to hand dominance. Dysphagia poststroke is associated with injury to the dominant representation.[88] Furthermore, patients with stroke who recover swallowing function have an increase in pharyngeal representation within the noninjured hemisphere, whereas those who remain with dysphagia show no change. This finding suggests that a potential treatment strategy for dysphagia would be to deliver excitatory rTMS to the noninjured pharyngeal motor cortex or to treat bilateral cortical regions with excitatory TMS. In a recent meta-analysis of 6 studies testing rTMS for the treatment of dysphagia poststroke, Liao and colleagues[89] found a large overall effect size of 1.24 (0.67–1.81, $P<.001$). High-frequency stimulation delivered bilaterally or to noninjured cortex produced superior improvement on swallowing outcomes in these studies. Brainstem strokes causing dysphagia, such as the lateral medullary syndrome, can also respond to cortical rTMS.[90] A recent study discovered that dysphagia following brainstem strokes was effectively treated with antidromic stimulation of the vagus nerve using high-frequency rTMS delivered over the left mastoid region.[91]

Neglect Syndrome

Hemispatial neglect, or neglect syndrome, is the failure to report, respond, or orient to stimuli presented contralateral to a brain lesion.[92] As many as 82% of patients with acute right hemisphere stroke show neglect syndrome, declining to about 30% to 50% in the chronic phase of recovery.[93,94] Unilateral spatial neglect is associated with longer rehabilitation length of stay with slower functional recovery and lower rate of discharge to home.[95,96] The clinical symptoms of neglect syndrome represent a dysfunction of the attentional-arousal system dominant in the right hemisphere. Attentional states involve complex frontoparietal networks in both hemispheres with strong inhibitory interhemispheric interconnectivity. An interhemispheric imbalance ensues following right cerebral injury leading to disinhibition and heightened excitability of left hemisphere networks, which then contributes to the rightward attentional bias.[97] The treatment of neglect syndrome has followed a similar scheme as for motor recovery by attempting to return hemispheric balance through neuromodulation using inhibitory stimulation to the left hemisphere, or less often with excitatory stimulation to the right hemisphere. Unlike motor recovery, the primary target site for stimulation is the posterior parietal cortex (PPC; P3 position of the 10–20 EEG system).

There are only a handful of studies testing rTMS in the treatment of stroke-related neglect syndrome. Koch and colleagues[98] reduced visual neglect and normalized hyperexcitable functional connectivity between PPC and M1 cortex by stimulating PPC with low-frequency (1 Hz) subthreshold rTMS. However, the clinical impact of left hemisphere downregulation using repeated sessions of low-frequency rTMS over 2 weeks in several clinical trials has only shown marginal improvement in attentional performance.[64,99,100] In contrast, just 1 session of continuous inhibitory cTBS improved perception of left-oriented targets for up to 32 hours in patients with right hemisphere stroke and neglect symptoms.[101] Further, 8 sessions of cTBS compared with sham or no treatment over 2 days improves target cancellation as well as scoring on the Catherine Bergego Scale, which measures neglect during basic functional activities.[102] A 2-week course of cTBS significantly improved scores on the behavioral inattention test up to 1 month posttreatment compared with sham, with an associated reduction in hyperexcitability of left frontoparietal circuits.[103] Presently, with only limited data, it seems that cTBS has the best potential to provide therapeutic neuromodulation for neglect syndrome.

Central Poststroke Pain

Central pain after stroke occurs in about 8% of cases and is associated with injury anywhere along the spinothalamic and thalamocortical pathways.[104,105] Central poststroke pain (CPSP) can respond to various oral medications, but outcomes are often limited by side effects or lack sufficient pain reduction.[106] There is now a growing interest in the use of motor cortex stimulation as a treatment of CPSP by implanted epidural electrode and pulse generator.[107] Studies overall show a 40% to 60% reduction in pain scores and a 50% overall success rate. Given the limited success and the risks of surgical electrode implantation, the use of TMS for management of poststroke pain has been explored.

Lefaucheur and colleagues[108,109] conducted early studies of rTMS to M1 cortex for neuropathic pain (including CPSP), showing that only high-frequency protocols achieved significant pain reduction, although patients with brainstem stroke do not respond as well as those with lesions in other locations. High-frequency stimulation over other cortical sites, such as premotor cortex, dorsolateral premotor cortex, S1 cortex, and supplementary motor cortex, do not reduce pain. Responders to M1 cortex stimulation have higher resting motor threshold and lower intracortical facilitation in the lesioned hemisphere. Following treatment, responders have an increase in intracortical facilitation.[110] Clinically, an improved warm detection threshold correlates with perceived pain reduction poststimulation, suggesting modulation of the thermoregulatory system, which includes somatosensory cortex, insula, and anterior cingulate gyrus.[111] This modulation via M1 cortex likely involves orthodromic corticofugal pathways to these structures as well as antidromic stimulation of the thalamocortical tracts.[110]

The problem with noninvasive stimulation for pain management after stroke is that the effects are transient and require repeated daily treatment. A single session can reduce pain for about 3 hours.[112] Five consecutive daily sessions can lead to prolonged pain reduction up to a month after the last treatment.[113] However, the impact of high-frequency rTMS for central neuropathic pain is modest at best. In the most recent Cochrane Review on noninvasive brain stimulation for chronic pain, pooled data for studies delivering a single session of high-frequency rTMS to motor cortex (N = 249) showed only a 12% reduction in pain, equating to a 0.77-point reduction on the visual analog scale, which fails to meet the threshold for minimally clinically important difference. There were insufficient data to suggest that multiple sessions improved overall outcomes and there was no evidence that the treatment reduced disability.[114] This analysis included a mix of pain causes. As such, patients with stroke and pain, especially those with cerebral lesions, likely have a better overall response to treatment.

SUMMARY

It is likely that TMS will be used for the clinical treatment of stroke and stroke-related impairments in the future. The anatomic target and stimulation parameters will likely vary for any clinical focus, be it weakness, pain, or cognitive or communicative dysfunction. Biomarkers may also be useful for identifying patients who will respond best, with a goal to enhance clinical decision making. Although not covered in this article because of limited available data, combination with drugs or specific types of therapeutic exercise may be necessary to achieve maximal response. Thus, there remain rich opportunities for research in noninvasive brain stimulation for stroke, and for many other conditions as well. Therapeutic TMS devices are already available on the market. Once clinicians identify optimal parameters for stroke treatment, the translation to common clinical use should be rapid.

REFERENCES

1. Winstein CJ, Wolf SL, Dromerick AW, et al. Effect of a task-oriented rehabilitation program on upper extremity recovery following motor stroke: the ICARE randomized clinical trial. JAMA 2016;315(6):571–81.
2. Duncan PW, Sullivan KJ, Behrman AL, et al. Body-weight-supported treadmill rehabilitation after stroke. N Engl J Med 2011;364(21):2026–36.
3. Krakauer JW, Cortés JC. A non-task-oriented approach based on high-dose playful movement exploration for rehabilitation of the upper limb early after stroke: a proposal. NeuroRehabilitation 2018;43(1):31–40.
4. Barker A, Jalinous R, Freeston I. Non-invasive magnetic stimulation of human motor cortex. Lancet 1985;1(8437):1106–7.
5. Ilmoniemi R, Virtanen J, Ruohonen J, et al. Neuronal responses to magnetic stimulation reveal cortical reactivity and connectivity. Neuroreport 1997;8: 3537–40.

6. Ilmoniemi R, Ruohonen J, Karhu J. Transcranial magnetic stimulation–a new tool for functional imaging of the brain. Crit Rev Biomed Eng 1999;27(3–5):241–84.

7. Ridding M, Rothwell J. Is there a future for therapeutic use of transcranial magnetic stimulation? Nat Rev Neurosci 2007;8(7):559–67.

8. Koponen L, Nieminen J, Ilmoniemi R. Multi-locus transcranial magnetic stimulation-theory and implementation. Brain Stimul 2018;11(4):849–55.

9. Deng Z, Lisanby S, Peterchev A. Electric field depth-focality tradeoff in transcranial magnetic stimulation: simulation comparison of 50 coil designs. Brain Stimul 2013;6(1):1–13.

10. Lontis E, Voigt M, Struijk J. Focality assessment in transcranial magnetic stimulation with double and cone coils. J Clin Neurophysiol 2006;23(5):462–71.

11. Roth Y, Zangen A, Hallett M. A coil design for transcranial magnetic stimulation of deep brain regions. J Clin Neurophysiol 2002;19(4):361–70.

12. Roth Y, Pell GS, Chistyakov AV, et al. Motor cortex activation by H-coil and figure-8 coil at different depths. Combined motor threshold and electric field distribution study. Clin Neurophysiol 2014;125:336–43.

13. Ilmoniemi R, Kicić D. Methodology for combined TMS and EEG. Brain Topogr 2010;22(4):233–48.

14. Bestmann S, Baudewig J, Siebner H, et al. BOLD MRI responses to repetitive TMS over human dorsal premotor cortex. Neuroimage 2005;28(1):22–9.

15. Paus T, Jech R, Thompson C, et al. Transcranial magnetic stimulation during positron emission tomography: a new method for studying connectivity of the human cerebral cortex. J Neurosci 1997;17(9):3178–84.

16. Näsi T, Mäki H, Kotilahti K, et al. Magnetic-stimulation-related physiological artifacts in hemodynamic near-infrared spectroscopy signals. PLoS One 2011;6(8): e24002.

17. Siebner H, Bergmann T, Bestmann S, et al. Consensus paper: combining transcranial stimulation with neuroimaging. Brain Stimul 2009;2(2):58–80.

18. Ruohonen J, Karhu J. Navigated transcranial magnetic stimulation. Neurophysiol Clin 2010;40(1):7–17.

19. Lioumis P, Kičić D, Savolainen P, et al. Reproducibility of TMS-evoked EEG responses. Hum Brain Mapp 2009;30(4):1387–96.

20. Casarotto S, Romero Lauro L, Bellina V, et al. EEG responses to TMS are sensitive to changes in the perturbation parameters and repeatable over time. PLoS One 2010;5(4):e10281.

21. Di Lazzaro V, Ziemann U, Lemon R. State of the art: physiology of transcranial motor cortex stimulation. Brain Stimul 2008;1(4):345–62.

22. Silvanto J, Lavie N, Walsh V. Double dissociation of V1 and V5/MT activity in visual awareness. Cereb Cortex 2005;15(11):1736–41.

23. Silvanto J. Transcranial magnetic stimulation and vision. Handb Clin Neurol 2013;116:655–69.

24. Brasil-Neto J, McShane L, Fuhr P, et al. Topographic mapping of the human motor cortex with magnetic stimulation: factors affecting accuracy and reproducibility. Electroencephalogr Clin Neurophysio 1992;85(1):9–16.

25. Amassian V, Eberle L, Maccabee P, et al. Modelling magnetic coil excitation of human cerebral cortex with a peripheral nerve immersed in a brain-shaped volume conductor: the significance of fiber bending in excitation. Electroencephalogr Clin Neurophysiol 1992;85(5):291–301.

26. Day B, Dressler D, Maertens de Noordhout A, et al. Electric and magnetic stimulation of human motor cortex: surface EMG and single motor unit responses. J Physiol 1989;412:449–73.

27. Maccabee P, Amassian V, Eberle L, et al. Magnetic coil stimulation of straight and bent amphibian and mammalian peripheral nerve in vitro: locus of excitation. J Physiol 1993;460:201–19.

28. Ruohonen J, Panizza M, Nilsson J, et al. Transverse-field activation mechanism in magnetic stimulation of peripheral nerves. Electroencephalogr Clin Neurophysiol 1996;101(2):167–74.

29. Di Lazzaro V, Profice P, Ranieri F, et al. I-wave origin and modulation. Brain Stimul 2012;5(4):512–25.

30. Di Lazzaro V, Ziemann U. The contribution of transcranial magnetic stimulation in the functional evaluation of microcircuits in human motor cortex. Front Neural Circuits 2013;7:18.

31. Chen R, Classen J, Gerloff C, et al. Depression of motor cortex excitability by low-frequency transcranial magnetic stimulation. Neurology 1997;48(5):1398–403.

32. Berardelli A, Inghilleri M, Rothwell J, et al. Facilitation of muscle evoked responses after repetitive cortical stimulation in man. Exp Brain Res 1998;122(1):79–84.

33. Siebner H, Rothwell J. Transcranial magnetic stimulation: new insights into representational cortical plasticity. Exp Brain Res 2003;148(11):1–16.

34. Platz T, Rothwell J. Brain stimulation and brain repair–rTMS: from animal experiment to clinical trials–what do we know? Restor Neurol Neurosci 2010;28(4):387–98.

35. Lefaucheur J, André-Obadia N, Antal A, et al. Evidence-based guidelines on the therapeutic use of repetitive transcranial magnetic stimulation (rTMS). Clin Neurophysiol 2014;125(11):2150–206.

36. Di Lazzaro V, Profice P, Pilato F, et al. The effects of motor cortex rTMS on corticospinal descending activity. Clin Neurophysiol 2010;121(4):464–73.

37. Wassermann E. Risk and safety of repetitive transcranial magnetic stimulation: report and suggested guidelines from the International Workshop on the Safety of Repetitive Transcranial Magnetic Stimulation, June 5-7, 1996. Electroencephalogr Clin Neurophysiol 1998;108(1):1–16.

38. Rossi S, Hallett M, Rossini P, et al, Safety of TMS Consensus Group. Safety, ethical considerations, and application guidelines for the use of transcranial magnetic stimulation in clinical practice and research. Clin Neurophysiol 2009;120(12):2008–39.

39. Dobek CE, Blumberger DM, Downar J, et al. Risk of seizures in transcranial magnetic stimulation: a clinical review to inform consent process focused on bupropion. Neuropsychiatr Dis Treat 2015;11:2975–87.

40. Nowak D, Grefkes C, Ameli M, et al. Interhemispheric competition after stroke: brain stimulation to enhance recovery of function of the affected hand. Neurorehabil Neural Repair 2009;23(7):641–56.

41. Dodd K, Nair V, Prabhakaran V. Role of the contralesional vs. ipsilesional hemisphere in stroke recovery. Front Hum Neurosci 2017;11:469.

42. Sanchez-Vives M, Nowak L, McCormick D. Cellular mechanisms of long-lasting adaptation in visual cortical neurons in vitro. J Neurosci 2000;20(11):4286–99.

43. Corti M, Patten C, Triggs W. Repetitive transcranial magnetic stimulation of motor cortex after stroke: a focused review. Am J Phys Med Rehabil 2012;91(3):254–70.

44. Kubis N. Non-invasive brain stimulation to enhance post-stroke recovery. Front Neural Circuits 2016;10:56.

45. Huang Y-Z, Edwards M, Rounis E, et al. Theta burst stimulation of the human motor cortex. Neuron 2005;45:201–6.

46. Suppa A, Huang Y, Funke K, et al. Ten years of theta burst stimulation in humans: established knowledge, unknowns and prospects. Brain Stimul 2016; 9(3):323–35.

47. Smith M, Stinear C. Transcranial magnetic stimulation (TMS) in stroke: ready for clinical practice? J Clin Neurosci 2016;31:10–4.

48. Zhang L, Xing G, Shuai S, et al. Low-frequency repetitive transcranial magnetic stimulation for stroke-induced upper limb motor deficit: a meta-analysis. Neural Plast 2017;2017:2758097.

49. Kondo T, Yamada N, Momosaki R, et al. Comparison of the effect of low-frequency repetitive transcranial magnetic stimulation with that of theta burst stimulation on upper limb motor function in poststroke patients. Biomed Res Int 2017;2017:4269435.

50. Suppa A, Ortu E, Zafar N, et al. Theta burst stimulation induces after-effects on contralateral primary motor cortex excitability in humans. J Physiol 2008; 586(18):4489–500.

51. Thickbroom G, Byrnes M, Edwards D, et al. Repetitive paired-pulse TMS at I-wave periodicity markedly increases corticospinal excitability: a new technique for modulating synaptic plasticity. Clin Neurophysiol 2006;117(1):61–6.

52. Hoogendam J, Ramakers G, Di Lazzaro V. Physiology of repetitive transcranial magnetic stimulation of the human brain. Brain Stimul 2010;3(2):95–118.

53. Hamada M, Hanajima R, Terao Y, et al. Quadro-pulse stimulation is more effective than paired-pulse stimulation for plasticity induction of the human motor cortex. Clin Neurophysiol 2007;118(12):2672–82.

54. Nakamura K, Groiss S, Hamada M, et al. Variability in response to quadripulse stimulation of the motor cortex. Brain Stimul 2016;9(6):859–66.

55. Gaynes BN, Lloyd SW, Lux L, et al. Repetitive transcranial magnetic stimulation for treatment-resistant depression: a systematic review and meta-analysis. J Clin Psychiatry 2014;75(5):477–89 [quiz: 489].

56. O'Reardon JP, Solvason HB, Janicak PG, et al. Efficacy and safety of transcranial magnetic stimulation in the acute treatment of major depression: a multisite randomized controlled trial. Biol Psychiatry 2007;62(11):1208–16.

57. Shen X, Liu M, Cheng Y, et al. Repetitive transcranial magnetic stimulation for the treatment of post-stroke depression: a systematic review and meta-analysis of randomized controlled clinical trials. J Affect Disord 2017;211:65–74.

58. Kwakkel G, Kollen BJ, van der Grond J, et al. Probability of regaining dexterity in the flaccid upper limb: impact of severity of paresis and time since onset in acute stroke. Stroke 2003;34(9):2181–6.

59. Perry J, Garrett M, Gronley JK, et al. Classification of walking handicap in the stroke population. Stroke 1995;26(6):982–9.

60. Fregni F, Boggio PS, Valle AC, et al. A sham-controlled trial of a 5-day course of repetitive transcranial magnetic stimulation of the unaffected hemisphere in stroke patients. Stroke 2006;37(8):2115–22.

61. Carey JR, Fregni F, Pascual-Leone A. rTMS combined with motor learning training in healthy subjects. Restor Neurol Neurosci 2006;24(3):191–9.

62. Swayne OB, Rothwell JC, Ward NS, et al. Stages of motor output reorganization after hemispheric stroke suggested by longitudinal studies of cortical physiology. Cereb Cortex 2008;18(8):1909–22.

63. Khedr EM, Abdel-Fadeil MR, Farghali A, et al. Role of 1 and 3 Hz repetitive transcranial magnetic stimulation on motor function recovery after acute ischaemic stroke. Eur J Neurol 2009;16(12):1323–30.

64. Kim BR, Chun MH, Kim DY, et al. Effect of high- and low-frequency repetitive transcranial magnetic stimulation on visuospatial neglect in patients with acute stroke: a double-blind, sham-controlled trial. Arch Phys Med Rehabil 2013;94: 803–7.

65. Malcolm MP, Triggs WJ, Light KE, et al. Repetitive transcranial magnetic stimulation as an adjunct to constraint-induced therapy: an exploratory randomized controlled trial. Am J Phys Med Rehabil 2007;86(9):707–15.

66. Ameli M, Grefkes C, Kemper F, et al. Differential effects of high-frequency repetitive transcranial magnetic stimulation over ipsilesional primary motor cortex in cortical and subcortical middle cerebral artery stroke. Ann Neurol 2009;66(3): 298–309.

67. Takeuchi N, Tada T, Toshima M, et al. Repetitive transcranial magnetic stimulation over bilateral hemispheres enhances motor function and training effect of paretic hand in patients after stroke. J Rehabil Med 2009;41(13):1049–54.

68. Yozbatiran N, Alonso-Alonso M, See J, et al. Safety and behavioral effects of high-frequency repetitive transcranial magnetic stimulation in stroke. Stroke 2009;40(1):309–12.

69. Khedr EM, Ahmed MA, Fathy N, et al. Therapeutic trial of repetitive transcranial magnetic stimulation after acute ischemic stroke. Neurology 2005;65(3):466–8.

70. Chang WH, Uhm KE, Shin YI, et al. Factors influencing the response to high-frequency repetitive transcranial magnetic stimulation in patients with subacute stroke. Restor Neurol Neurosci 2016;34(5):747–55.

71. Emara TH, Moustafa RR, Elnahas NM, et al. Repetitive transcranial magnetic stimulation at 1Hz and 5Hz produces sustained improvement in motor function and disability after ischaemic stroke. Eur J Neurol 2010;17(9):1203–9.

72. Takeuchi N, Tada T, Toshima M, et al. Inhibition of the unaffected motor cortex by 1 Hz repetitive transcranical magnetic stimulation enhances motor performance and training effect of the paretic hand in patients with chronic stroke. J Rehabil Med 2008;40(4):298–303.

73. Harvey RL, Edwards D, Dunning K, et al. Randomized sham-controlled trial of navigated repetitive transcranial magnetic stimulation for motor recovery in stroke: the NICHE trial. Stroke 2018;49(9):2138–46.

74. Cha HG, Kim MK. Effects of strengthening exercise integrated repetitive transcranial magnetic stimulation on motor function recovery in subacute stroke patients: a randomized controlled trial. Technol Health Care 2017;25(3):521–9.

75. Ji S-G, Kim M-K. The effect of repetitive transcranial magnetic stimulation on the gait of acute stroke patients. Journal of Magnetics 2015;20(2):129–32.

76. Ji S-G, Shin Y-J, Kim M-K. The effects of repetitive transcranial magnetic stimulation on balance ability in acute stroke patients. J Korean Soc Phys Med 2016; 11(3):11–7.

77. Wang RY, Tseng HY, Liao KK, et al. rTMS combined with task-oriented training to improve symmetry of interhemispheric corticomotor excitability and gait performance after stroke: a randomized trial. Neurorehabil Neural Repair 2012;26(3): 222–30.

78. Chieffo R, De Prezzo S, Houdayer E, et al. Deep repetitive transcranial magnetic stimulation with H-coil on lower limb motor function in chronic stroke: a pilot study. Arch Phys Med Rehabil 2014;95(6):1141–7.

79. Kakuda W, Abo M, Nakayama Y, et al. High-frequency rTMS using a double cone coil for gait disturbance. Acta Neurol Scand 2013;128(2):100–6.
80. Talelli P, Greenwood RJ, Rothwell JC. Exploring theta burst stimulation as an intervention to improve motor recovery in chronic stroke. Clin Neurophysiol 2007;118(2):333–42.
81. Talelli P, Wallace A, Dileone M, et al. Theta burst stimulation in the rehabilitation of the upper limb: a semirandomized, placebo-controlled trial in chronic stroke patients. Neurorehabil Neural Repair 2012;26(8):976–87.
82. Long H, Wang H, Zhao C, et al. Effects of combining high- and low-frequency repetitive transcranial magnetic stimulation on upper limb hemiparesis in the early phase of stroke. Restor Neurol Neurosci 2018;36(1):21–30.
83. Sasaki N, Kakuda W, Abo M. Bilateral high- and low-frequency rTMS in acute stroke patients with hemiparesis: a comparative study with unilateral high-frequency rTMS. Brain Inj 2014;28(13–14):1682–6.
84. Sung WH, Wang CP, Chou CL, et al. Efficacy of coupling inhibitory and facilitatory repetitive transcranial magnetic stimulation to enhance motor recovery in hemiplegic stroke patients. Stroke 2013;44(5):1375–82.
85. Hao Z, Wang D, Zeng Y, et al. Repetitive transcranial magnetic stimulation for improving function after stroke. Cochrane Database Syst Rev 2013;(5):CD008862.
86. Ling HM, Tao T, Xu J, et al. Effects of repetitive transcranial magnetic stimulation on upper limb motor function in patients with stroke: a meta analysis. Zhanghua Y Xue Z Zhi 2017;97:3739–45.
87. Winstein CJ, Stein J, Arena R, et al. Guidelines for adult stroke rehabilitation and recovery. A guideline for healthcare professionals from the American Heart Association/American Stroke Association. Stroke 2016;47(6):e98–169.
88. Hamdy S, Aziz Q, Rothwell JC, et al. The cortical topography of human swallowing musculature in health and disease. Nat Med 1996;2(11):1217–24.
89. Liao X, Xing G, Guo Z, et al. Repetitive transcranial magnetic stimulation as an alternative therapy for dysphagia after stroke: a systematic review and meta-analysis. Clin Rehabil 2017;31(3):289–98.
90. Khedr EM, Abo-Elfetoh N. Therapeutic role of rTMS on recovery of dysphagia in patients with lateral medullary syndrome and brainstem infarction. J Neurol Neurosurg Psychiatry 2010;81:495–9.
91. Lin WS, Chou CL, Chang MH, et al. Vagus nerve magnetic modulation facilitates dysphagia recovery in patients with stroke involving the brainstem – a proof of concept study. Brain Stimul 2018;11:264–70.
92. Heilman KM, Watson RT, Valenstein E. Neglect and related disorders. In: Heilman KM, Valenstein E, editors. Clinical neuropsychology. 3rd edition. New York: Oxford University Press; 1993. p. 279–336.
93. Baxbaum LJ, Ferraro MK, Veramonti T, et al. Hemispatial neglect: subtypes, neuroanatomy, and disability. Neurology 2004;62:749–56.
94. Stone SP, Halliagan PW, Greenwood RJ. The incidence of neglect phenomena and related disorders in patients with an acute right or left hemisphere stroke. Age Ageing 1993;22:46–52.
95. Chen P, Hreha K, Kong Y, et al. Impact of spatial neglect on stroke rehabilitation: evidence from the setting of an impatient rehabilitation facility. Arch Phys Med Rehabil 2015;96:1458–66.
96. Gillen R, Tennen H, McKee T. Unilateral spatial neglect: relation to rehabilitation outcomes in patients with right hemisphere stroke. Arch Phys Med Rehabil 2005;86:763–7.

97. Hesse MD, Sparing R, Fink GR. Ameliorating spatial neglect with non-invasive brain stimulation: from pathophysiological concepts to novel treatment strategies. Neuropsychol Rehabil 2011;21:676–702.
98. Koch G, Oliveri M, Cheeran B, et al. Hyperexcitability of parietal-motor functional connections for the intact left-hemisphere in neglect patients. Brain 2008;131: 3147–55.
99. Song W, Du B, Xu Q, et al. Low-frequency transcranial magnetic stimulation for visual spatial neglect: a pilot study. J Rehabil Med 2009;41:162–5.
100. Yang NYH, Fong KNK, Li-Tsang CWP, et al. Effects of repetitive transcranial magnetic stimulation combined with sensory cueing on unilateral neglect in subacute patients with right hemispheric stroke: a randomized controlled study. Clin Rehabil 2017;31:1154–63.
101. Nyffeler T, Cazzoli D, Hess CW, et al. One session of repeated parietal theta burst stimulation trains induces long-lasting improvement of visual neglect. Stroke 2009;40:2791–6.
102. Cazzoli D, Muri RM, Schumacher R, et al. Theta burst stimulation reduces disability during the activities of daily living in spatial neglect. Brain 2012;135: 3426–9.
103. Koch G, Bonni S, Giacobbe V, et al. Theta-burst stimulation of the left hemisphere accelerates recovery of hemispatial neglect. Neurology 2012;78:24–30.
104. Andersen G, Vestergaard K, Ingeman-Neilsen M, et al. Incidence of central post stroke pain. Pain 1995;61:187–93.
105. Cassinari V, Pagni CA. Central pain. A neurological survey. Cambridge (United Kingdom): Harvard University Press; 1969.
106. Harvey RL. Central poststroke pain syndrome. Top Stroke Rehabil 2010;17: 163–72.
107. Hosomi B, Seymour B, Saitoh Y. Modulating the pain network–neurostimulation for central poststroke pain. Nat Rev Neurol 2015;11:290–9.
108. Lefaucheur JP, Drouot X, Keravel Y, et al. Pain relief induced by repetitive transcranial magnetic stimulation of precentral cortex. Neuroreport 2001;12(13): 2963–5.
109. Lefaucheur JP, Drouot X, Menard-Lefaucheur I, et al. Neurogenic pain relief by repetitive transcranial magnetic cortical stimulation depends on the origin and the site of pain. J Neurol Neurosurg Psychiatry 2004;75(4):612–6.
110. Hosomi K, Kishima H, Oshino S, et al. Cortical excitability changes after high-frequency repetitive transcranial magnetic stimulation for central poststroke pain. Pain 2013;154(8):1352–7.
111. Hasan M, Whiteley J, Bresnahan R, et al. Somatosensory change and pain relief induced by repetitive transcranial magnetic stimulation in patients with central poststroke pain. Neuromodulation 2014;17(8):731–6 [discussion: 736].
112. Hirayama A, Saitoh Y, Kishima H, et al. Reduction of intractable deafferentation pain by navigation-guided repetitive transcranial magnetic stimulation of the primary motor cortex. Pain 2006;122(1–2):22–7.
113. Jin Y, Xing G, Li G, et al. High frequency repetitive transcranial magnetic stimulation therapy for chronic neuropathic pain: a meta-analysis. Pain Physician 2015;18(6):E1029–46.
114. O'Connell NE, Marston L, Spencer S, et al. Non-invasive brain stimulation techniques for chronic pain. Cochrane Database Syst Rev 2018;(4):CD008208.

Spinal Cord Epidural Stimulation for Lower Limb Motor Function Recovery in Individuals with Motor Complete Spinal Cord Injury

Enrico Rejc, PhD[a,b,*], Claudia A. Angeli, PhD[a,c]

KEYWORDS

- Spinal cord injury • Epidural stimulation • Activity-based training
- Spinal motor learning • Rehabilitation • Neuromodulation

KEY POINTS

- Spinal cord epidural stimulation can neuromodulate the human spinal circuitry controlling posture and locomotion, which remains most often intact below the level of injury, by primarily recruiting dorsal root fibers carrying somatosensory information.
- Spinal cord epidural stimulation, sensory feedback, and clinically undetected, residual volitional descending input can synergistically contribute to motor function recovery after chronic, motor complete spinal cord injury.
- The selection of spinal cord epidural stimulation parameters and characteristics of activity-based training crucially influence motor function recovery.
- Future studies with a larger number of individuals and advanced epidural stimulation technology are needed to better understand the motor recovery potential after severe spinal cord injury.

 Video content accompanies this article at http://www.pmr.theclinics.com/.

INTRODUCTION

Severe spinal cord injury (SCI) dramatically impairs motor function, leading also to serious health-related complications in the affected individuals. Activity-based therapies for motor function recovery are focused on activating the neuromuscular system

Disclosure Statement: The authors have nothing to disclose.
[a] Kentucky Spinal Cord Injury Research Center, University of Louisville, 220 Abraham Flexner Way, Louisville, KY 40202, USA; [b] Department of Neurological Surgery, University of Louisville, Louisville, KY, USA; [c] Frazier Rehab Institute, KentuckyOne Health, 220 Abraham Flexner Way, Louisville, KY 40202, USA
* Corresponding author. Kentucky Spinal Cord Injury Research Center, University of Louisville, 220 Abraham Flexner Way, Louisville, KY 40202.
E-mail addresses: enrico.rejc@louisville.edu; EnricoRejc@KentuckyOneHealth.org

Phys Med Rehabil Clin N Am 30 (2019) 337–354
https://doi.org/10.1016/j.pmr.2018.12.009
1047-9651/19/© 2018 Elsevier Inc. All rights reserved.

below the level of injury, because in most cases the spinal circuitry controlling posture and locomotion remains intact. This approach can promote positive functional adaptations even years after an incomplete SCI.[1,2] On the other hand, individuals with more complete and chronic injuries have poor prognosis for recovery of standing, stepping, and voluntary leg movements.[3,4]

In the last decade, different types of spinal cord stimulation (ie, lumbosacral spinal cord epidural stimulation [scES], transcutaneous stimulation, magnetic stimulation) have been tested in humans with the goal of promoting lower limb motor function recovery after severe SCI,[5–7] and other stimulation approaches (ie, intraspinal microstimulation[8]) are in the process of being translated to humans. This review focuses on scES strategies that, combined with activity-based training, have shown promising results in terms of lower limb motor function recovery after chronic, clinically motor complete SCI in humans.

SPINAL CORD CHARACTERISTICS UNDERLYING SPINAL STIMULATION- AND TRAINING-INDUCED MOTOR RECOVERY AFTER SPINAL CORD INJURY

Spinal cord stimulation and activity-based training aim at capitalizing on the human spinal cord sensory-motor potential that still persists after chronic, clinically complete SCI. In particular, (i) automaticity, (ii) residual supraspinal connections to the spinal circuitry, and (iii) plasticity are briefly discussed in this section.

Automaticity of the Spinal Circuitry Controlling Posture and Locomotion

Lumbosacral spinal circuitry controlling posture and locomotion maintains the capability to generate relatively complex activation patterns following the disruption of supraspinal input.[9,10] For example, it preserves the potential to generate oscillating coordinated motor patterns, which can be modulated by peripheral sensory information received from the spinal cord, although in a modified manner compared with an intact system. Individuals with no detectable supraspinal input to the lumbosacral spinal circuitry can generate electromyographic (EMG) locomotor pattern when stepping on a treadmill with body weight support (BWS) and manual assistance.[11,12] EMG pattern during assisted stepping may vary across SCI individuals,[11] conceivably because of the intrinsic characteristics of the lesion and following reorganization of the spinal circuitry.[13–15] Importantly, changes in sensory information (ie, amount of body weight support; treadmill speed) can modulate EMG locomotor pattern, highlighting the potential of sensory information received by the lumbosacral spinal circuitry to control motor pattern.[16,17]

Residual Supraspinal Connectivity to the Spinal Circuitry after Motor Complete Spinal Cord Injury

In an intact nervous system, supraspinal input to the spinal circuitry is one of the main components of the automaticity of motor control. In particular, supraspinal input provides nonspecific tonic drive that optimizes the spinal circuitry state of excitability to perform a motor task (ie, walking or standing).[9] After a motor complete SCI, the prevailing view is that the loss of supraspinal tonic drive to the spinal circuitry disrupts its sustainable excitability,[11] leading to the inability to stand and step. It also appears that the excitability level of human lumbosacral spinal circuitry is more depressed after severe SCI compared with other mammals[18]; this would contribute to explain why some animal models (ie, cats) can recover full weight-bearing standing and stepping, whereas humans do not show the same recovery capability. However, it is important to note that most of the clinically complete SCI are not anatomically complete.[19] In addition, it is not rare to detect EMG activity from the paralyzed leg muscles in response to volitional movement attempts, with or without the concurrent volitional activation of muscles above the level of injury, in individuals classified as clinically motor complete (ie, motor discomplete SCI).[20–22] The importance of residual nondetectable and/or nonfunctional descending input for motor recovery using spinal stimulation is discussed later in dedicated sections of this article.

Training-Induced Plasticity

Activity-based training is crucial to modulate the properties of spinal circuitry and improve motor recovery after SCI.[23–25] Factors and mechanisms underlying training-induced functional improvements after complete SCI have been extensively studied in animal models, focusing on behavioral changes as well as physiological and biochemical adaptations occurring in the spinal cord below the level of injury.[26–28] Training-induced plasticity is dependent on the training volume[29]; however, their relationship is not well detailed yet.[18] Importantly, the motor task that is repetitively practiced affects the characteristics of training-induced neural plasticity, leading to task-specific adaptations that can also affect the ability of the spinal cord to learn novel motor tasks.[30,31] In addition, some level of variability in the trained motor pattern was found effective for enhancing motor recovery.[32,33] Training-induced plasticity not only targets the spinal circuitry below the level of injury but also can modulate the supraspinal structures and their connections to the spinal circuitry.[34,35]

Earlier Applications of Spinal Cord Epidural Stimulation for Pain Management and Functional Improvement in Motor Disorders

ScES has been used for more than 40 years in individuals with different neurological conditions. In the 1960s, scES had been investigated as a clinical application for pain control, with some initial success for reduction of chronic pain in 42% of the cases.[36] Also, improvements in motor function that were initially observed in the 1970s in one individual with multiple sclerosis[37,38] were subsequently confirmed in other patients with the same condition[39] as well as in other motor disorders (ie, spasticity).[40–44] Interestingly, most of these studies already reported empirical evidence supporting the view that the appropriate selection of scES parameters (site and/or electrode configuration, stimulation frequency, and amplitude) was critical for promoting the desired neuromodulation, and that these parameters were substantially individual-specific. Initial experiments performed to better understand the scES-induced neurophysiological adaptations in the spinal circuitry reported controversial results.[45,46] Subsequently, more comprehensive investigations in individuals with complete and incomplete SCI highlighted the complexity of the interaction between scES and characteristics of spinal cord neuromodulation. In particular, it was demonstrated that the effects of scES on spasticity was dependent on location, frequency, and voltage of scES,[47,48] and that either facilitation or inhibition of spinal reflex activity can be promoted by scES depending on the parameters applied.[49]

Spinal Cord Epidural Stimulation Can Access and Neuromodulate the Spinal Circuitry Controlling Posture and Locomotion After Severe Spinal Cord Injury

The mechanisms underlying the enhancement of spinal circuitry for motor pattern generation by scES are not yet completely understood. However, neurophysiological recordings[50–57] as well as computational models[58,59] suggest that scES primarily recruits large myelinated fibers associated with somatosensory information, and particularly with proprioceptive and cutaneous feedback circuits, at their entry into the spinal cord as well as along the longitudinal portions of the fiber trajectories, altering the excitability of spinal circuits involved in motor pattern generation. In particular, proprioceptive, muscle spindle feedback circuits were found to be primarily involved in the modulation of locomotor pattern promoted by scES.[56,57] Regarding the pathways that can be modulated by scES, it is important to recognize the role of both complex spinal neural connections and stimulation parameters. For example, previous studies reported that most muscles are innervated by several spinal segments, which can be interconnected via ascending or descending projections, and that the motoneurons network appears to be broadly spaced over wide regions of the spinal cord.[60–62] Also, extensive divergence of a single Ia fiber from each muscle spindle showed extensive synaptic connectivity to the homonymous motor pools as well as to synergists and, indirectly, to antagonistic motor pools through Ia inhibitory interneurons.[63] Hence, scES may impact many different sensory-motor pathways simultaneously, even if a relatively localized stimulation is applied.[64] Moreover, stimulation frequency, amplitude, and site (electrode configuration) play a crucial role in determining extent and proportion of the modulation of these pathways.[65]

Stimulation Frequency and Amplitude

Early research showed that lumbosacral scES has the potential to access the human spinal circuitry and induce the generation of lower limb motor patterns.[66] This pivotal research demonstrated that steplike movements could be induced in paraplegic individuals lying supine by applying a tonic electrical drive to the lumbosacral spinal cord via 2 active electrodes of a quadripolar array, selecting frequencies between 25 and 60 Hz and amplitudes well above motor threshold. Further studies suggested that, with high stimulation amplitudes, frequencies between 5 and 15 Hz were optimal to induce a lower limb tonic extensor pattern,[67] whereas frequencies between 25 and 50 Hz were optimal for inducing rhythmic activation patterns.[68–70] The fact that either a tonic extensor pattern or a rhythmic pattern could be elicited using lower or higher stimulation frequencies in a group of SCI individuals lying supine, without any change in stimulation site and intensity (**Fig. 1**), was interpreted as different frequencies would access different inhibitory and/or excitatory pathways within spinal networks to elicit different EMG patterns.[67]

On the other hand, when lower (near-motor threshold) stimulation amplitudes were applied to motor complete SCI individuals in the upright position bearing full body weight, higher stimulation frequencies (ie, 25–60 Hz) could promote overall continuous (ie, nonrhythmic) EMG patterns.[71] In this condition, higher stimulation frequencies also led to greater variability of the evoked responses to scES, possibly because of the progressive integration of additional afferent inputs through the greater involvement of interneurons.[69,71,72]

In an effort to better understand the neuromodulatory role of scES amplitude, a series of experiments was performed with motor complete SCI individuals in the supine position. EMG outcomes suggested that lower scES amplitudes resulted in initial recruitment of the lower threshold afferent structures, whereas with higher amplitudes more efferent volleys are involved, precluding the response that may have been driven by the afferent pathways and possibly leading to the activation of motoneurons and/or anterior roots.[64]

Electrode Configuration

Stimulation site and electrodes configuration have important implications for both topographical and functional organization of the activation pattern induced or facilitated by scES. In SCI individuals lying supine, localized, low-frequency (2 Hz) scES

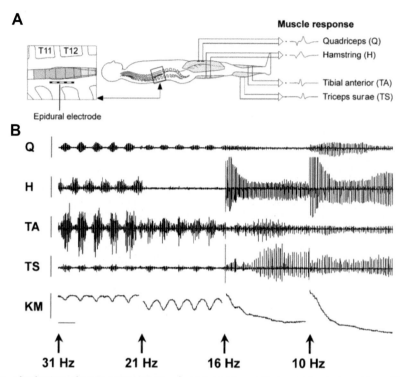

Fig. 1. Rhythmic and tonic EMG activity of paralyzed lower limb muscles induced by scES. (*A*) Outline of the clinical assessment design. The subjects were placed in the supine position; pairs of surface EMG electrodes were placed over the bellies of the lower limb muscle groups. The approximate scES electrode position is also reported. (*B*) EMG recordings obtained from the lower limb muscle groups during spinal cord stimulation at frequencies of 31 and 21 Hz (rhythmic activity) as compared with 16 and 10 Hz (tonic activity), while stimulation site and strength (10 V) remained constant. Vertical markers: 500 μV (Q, H, TA, TS); 45° (KM, knee movement, assessed by a goniometer). Horizontal marker: 1 second. (*Adapted from* Jilge B, Minassian K, Rattay F, et al. Initiating extension of the lower limbs in subjects with complete spinal cord injury by epidural lumbar cord stimulation. Exp Brain Res 2004;154(3):310–4; with permission.)

of rostral and caudal areas of lumbosacral spinal cord resulted in selective topographical recruitment of proximal and distal leg muscles, respectively,[64] in agreement with the anatomy and myotomal maps of the spinal cord and lumbosacral roots.[61,73,74] On the other hand, both proximal and distal muscles were recruited in a non-location-specific manner when a wide electrode field was applied. Side-specific activation modulation can also be achieved by modifying the mediolateral positioning of the electrode with respect to the spinal cord, as shown in rats with complete spinal injuries[59] and observed via neurophysiologic recordings during surgical implantation of the scES electrode array in humans.[75]

The stimulation site is also relevant for the functional characteristics of motor output generated using scES. For example, some evidence suggested that L2 spinal level is most responsive to epidural stimulation for inducing locomotor-like activity in humans (and also in rats).[66,76] On the other hand, electrode configurations with the cathode (active electrode) positioned in the caudal area of the lumbosacral spinal cord, and more caudal than the anode, were considered more effective for generating lower limb extensor pattern.[58,67,77]

SPINAL CORD EPIDURAL STIMULATION, SENSORY FEEDBACK, AND RESIDUAL VOLITIONAL DESCENDING INPUT: SYNERGIC CONTRIBUTION FOR MOTOR FUNCTION RECOVERY AFTER SPINAL CORD INJURY

Decades of work on animal models with complete SCI initially suggested to apply scES with the goal of modulating the excitability of spinal circuitry, mimicking the tonic supraspinal drive lost after SCI, so that sensory information from lower limbs could serve as a source of control for generating appropriate motor patterns during standing and stepping.[9] In addition, the serendipitous findings related to the reenabling of volitional lower limb movements using scES led to further efforts aimed at investigating and improving volitional control of non-weight-bearing motor tasks. Under this condition, the integration of somatosensory and residual descending inputs to the spinal circuitry contributes to motor control, with the descending input playing a primary role for different aspects, such as movement initiation and cessation. Interestingly, it was observed that volitional input can modulate motor patterns also during weight-bearing standing and assisted stepping; ongoing studies are investigating the consistent integration of residual volitional descending input during standing and stepping practice with scES. In all these conditions, the selection of scES parameters and activity-based training crucially influence the extent and characteristics of motor recovery.

Spinal Cord Epidural Stimulation Reenabled Standing Using Sensory Feedback as a Source of Control

When an individual with motor complete SCI is assisted (ie, by trainers) to perform a sitting to standing transition, lower limb EMG activity is usually observed during the transition phase (**Fig. 2**A). Conversely, when the individual achieves a stable upright position, which is maintained via external assistance, EMG activity of lower limb muscles is generally negligible or absent (see **Fig. 2**B), being similar to that recorded during sitting.[78]

scES applied for reenabling full weight-bearing standing in clinically motor complete SCI individuals did not impose directly lower limb motor responses by stimulating the spinal cord at high intensities; conversely, EMG pattern generation was promoted by the sensory feedback projected to the spinal circuitry, the physiologic state of which was properly modulated by scES.[71] In particular, scES applied in sitting did not induce any lower limb movement or relevant muscle activation (see **Fig. 2**C). However, the sensory information related to the change in body position from sitting to standing significantly modulated EMG, leading to the generation of activation patterns sufficient for standing without any change in scES parameters. The proposed approach allowed 2 sensory and motor complete SCI individuals to achieve full weight-bearing standing without any external assistance, using their upper limbs for assisting balance control (see **Fig. 2**D). Two other motor complete SCI individuals also needed external hip extension facilitation for achieving standing.[71] Independent standing was promoted by an overall continuous EMG pattern of the lower limb muscles that resulted in constant level of ground reaction forces.

Spinal Cord Epidural Stimulation Facilitated Assisted Stepping Using Sensory Feedback as a Source of Control

Individuals with clinically complete SCI show substantial variability in the activation pattern generated during assisted stepping. However, one of the common patterns

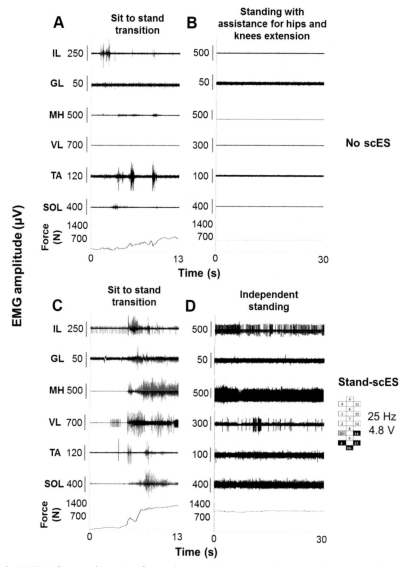

Fig. 2. EMG and ground reaction forces during sitting-to-standing transition and during standing. Time course of EMG activity and ground reaction forces recorded from a clinically sensory and motor complete SCI individual during sitting-to-standing transition and during stable standing without scES (*A* and *B*, respectively) and with scES optimized for standing (*C* and *D*, respectively). Stimulation frequency, amplitude, and electrode configuration (cathodes in black; anodes in gray; and nonactive in white) are reported. IL, iliopsoas; GL, gluteus maximus; MH, medial hamstring; SOL, soleus; TA, tibialis anterior; VL, vastus lateralis. (*From* Krames E, Peckham PH, Rezai AR. Neuromodulation: comprehensive textbook of principles, technologies, and therapies. 2nd edition. London: Academic Press is an imprint of Elsevier; 2018: ScienceDirect. Available at: https://www.sciencedirect.com/science/book/9780128053539; with permission.)

results in minimal EMG activity limited to very few muscles, regardless of variations in speed and load.[11] In one SCI individual who showed these characteristics, the application of scES during assisted stepping on a treadmill with BWS using below motor threshold stimulation amplitude resulted in the generation of EMG bursts timed to the step cycle (**Fig. 3**).[5]

This finding was interpreted as scES increased the overall excitability level of the spinal networks, which was not sufficient to interpret sensory information during manually facilitated stepping without stimulation. The ability of the spinal networks to interpret sensory information (ie, load, speed, direction) during stepping has been demonstrated in different human[12,17] and animal models.[27,57,79–81] scES can also modulate and

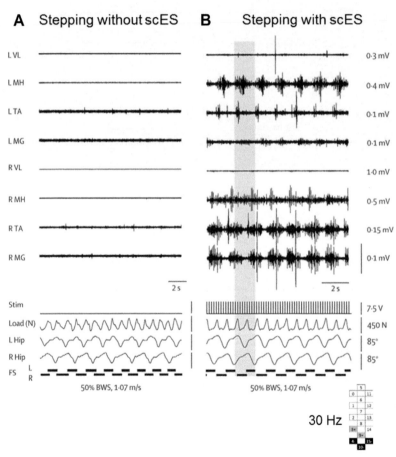

Fig. 3. EMG activity of lower limb muscles during assisted stepping on a treadmill with BWS without (A) and with (B) scES. The gray shaded area shows one full step of the right leg. BWS, treadmill speed, stimulation frequency, and electrode configuration (cathodes in black; anodes in gray; and nonactive in white) are reported at the bottom of the figure. BWS, body weight support; FS, footswitches; L, left; L Hip, left hip sagittal joint angle; Load, load cell reading; MG, medial gastrocnemius; R, right; R Hip, right hip sagittal joint angle; Stim, stimulation intensity. (*Adapted from* Harkema S, Gerasimenko Y, Hodes J, et al. Effect of epidural stimulation of the lumbosacral spinal cord on voluntary movement, standing, and assisted stepping after motor complete paraplegia: a case study. Lancet 2011;377(9781):1944; with permission.)

"change the timing of efferent motor patterns" during assisted stepping on a treadmill with BWS when higher (above motor threshold) scES amplitudes and frequencies (ie, 30 Hz) are applied.[82] However, when higher amplitudes were maintained and lower frequencies (ie, those that induced extensor tonic pattern in supine) were applied, the scES-induced tonic extensor motor pattern of the lower limb was not modulated by the addition of stepping sensory information (ie, remained tonic throughout the step cycle). These evidences suggest that scES amplitudes high enough to directly elicit a motor pattern may mask and/or alter the potential of the spinal networks to organize the motor pattern generation using sensory feedback as a source of control.

Spinal Cord Epidural Stimulation Reenabled Volitional Lower Limb Motor Control Under Non-Weight-Bearing Conditions

A surprising observation of volitional lower extremity movement in an individual with motor complete SCI following stand training with scES shifted the dogma of epidural stimulation as a driver of specific motor patterns to enabling innate patterns to emerge.[5] Because of the long training period before the discovery of the ability to generate volitional movements, it was speculated that strengthening of residual supraspinal influence and/or plasticity in descending pathways (ie, sprouting) may have resulted in this newfound ability. However, 3 additional individuals diagnosed with motor complete injuries were later shown to be able to volitionally perform leg movements in the presence of subthreshold levels of scES before the occurrence of any training.[55] The level of control over the movement in the presence of scES was notable, because it included timing (linked to visual and auditory cues) and grade effort.[55,83] More recently, an SCI individual with chronic discomplete injury was able to volitionally initiate, terminate, and modulate rhythmic locomotor-like activity of one limb, which was suspended using a fabric support, while being in a side-lying position.[83] Similar findings were reported by Gerasimenko and colleagues[6] while applying transcutaneous electrical stimulation of the spinal cord in clinically motor complete SCI individuals positioned side lying on a gravity-neutral apparatus. These observations support the hypothesis that scES modulates the excitability of spinal circuitry, allowing the supraspinal input to travel across small and dormant fibers, engaging the appropriate spinal networks to generate the desired motor pattern. The "augmenting" effect of submotor threshold scES on supraspinal input was experimentally demonstrated in a rat model[84]; in fact, the amplitude of motor potentials evoked from cortical stimulation was substantially increased in the presence of timed scES delivered at 90% of motor threshold. This last study also provides evidence that the site of convergence of descending input and spinal afferents is conceivably the cervical spinal cord.

Volitional Motor Pattern Modulation During Standing and Assisted Stepping with Spinal Cord Epidural Stimulation

The integration of sensory and supraspinal signals by the spinal circuitry in motor complete SCI individuals using scES was further demonstrated in their ability to intentionally modulate the motor pattern generated during standing and assisted stepping. For example, starting from a condition of stable standing with independence of knee extension and facilitation (by elastic cords) for hip extension, 2 research participants were able to volitionally decrease the lower limb muscle activation without any change in stimulation parameters (**Fig. 4**A), achieving a controlled lower limb flexion limited by the elastic cords positioned at the hips and knees (Video 1). When the squatted position was reached, they were able to volitionally promote the reemergence of an activation pattern that led to extension and standing. This observation may suggest that residual descending inhibitory input can be preserved after severe SCI[20] and can be volitionally accessed while scES is applied for facilitating standing.

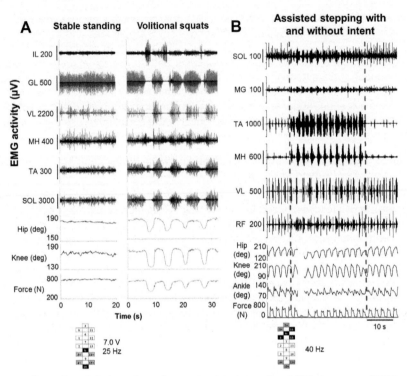

Fig. 4. Volitional modulation of standing and assisted stepping. (*A*) Time course of EMG activity, hip and knee angle, and ground reaction forces recorded from a clinically motor complete SCI individual during stable standing with scES and during volitional squats. The lower limb flexion was limited by elastic cords positioned at hips and knees during squatting (see Video 1). (*B*) Time course of EMG activity, lower limb kinematics, and ground reaction forces recorded from a clinically motor and sensory complete SCI individual during assisted stepping on a treadmill with scES. The recording within the dashed lines shows the stepping period during which the subject is consciously thinking about stepping and trying to volitionally contribute to each step. Stimulation frequency, amplitude, and electrode configuration (cathodes in black; anodes in gray; and nonactive in white) are reported at the bottom of the figure. IL, iliopsoas; RF, rectus femoris; SOL, soleus. ([*B*] *Adapted from* Angeli CA, Edgerton VR, Gerasimenko YP, et al. Altering spinal cord excitability enables voluntary movements after chronic complete paralysis in humans. Brain 2014;137(Pt 5):1394–409; with permission.)

Similarly, Angeli and colleagues[55] demonstrated that 2 participants were able to change timing and amplitude of motor output (primarily of flexor muscles) during assisted stepping on a treadmill while consciously trying to contribute to the step cycle (see **Fig. 4**B). Such modulation was not present in the absence of scES. A more recent report showed that scES also enabled a motor discomplete SCI individual to volitionally initiate and control steplike movements while being in an upright position, overground, with body weight supported by a harness.[83]

Epidural Stimulation Strategies and Parameters

Tonic spinal cord epidural stimulation

A series of observations and experiments showed that the appropriate selection of tonic scES parameters is crucial to facilitate the generation of effective motor patterns and that, in the vast majority of the cases, these parameters are individual and task specific.[65,71] In particular, one of the goals for the selection of scES parameters is an appropriate activation level of the lower limb muscles (considering proximal and distal muscles; left and right side; extensors and flexors) during the motor task execution. Other important objectives are the facilitation of a rhythmic or continuous motor pattern, and maximizing the influence of descending input for lower limb motor pattern modulation.

As reported above, electrode configuration, stimulation amplitude, and frequency are interrelated variables affecting the motor pattern; to date, there are no available algorithms or procedures that suggest the exact set of parameters to be applied in individuals with SCI. However, a proposed approach for selecting a subset of electrode configurations (among the $\sim 4.3 \times 10^7$ available in a 16-electrode array) to be tested for functional recovery is based on the topographical recruitment knowledge (ie, focusing more on either the caudal or the rostral portion of the electrode array to increase the excitability of distal or proximal muscles' motoneuron pools, respectively) as well as on the individualized map of motor pools activation. In addition, the prevailing functional facilitation of different stimulation sites (ie, spinal level L2 for rhythmic activity[66,76]; caudal area of the lumbosacral spinal cord for lower limb extensor pattern[58,67,77]) should be also considered.

The use of multiple interleaving programs (up to 4 in the Medtronic Restore ADVANCED stimulatior using the 5-6-5 Specify electrode array [Medtronic, Minneapolis, MN, USA]; see, for example, research participant A53 in Ref.[71]) can represent an important advantage compared with the use of a single program, because it allows access to different locations of the spinal circuitry with different voltages. This approach is used in ongoing studies from the authors' laboratory and has contributed to an overall improvement in functional outcomes; however, future studies are needed to better understand its neuromodulatory mechanisms. Similarly, multisite spinal stimulation was shown more effective than single site for promoting stepping motor pattern in animal and in vitro models[85,86] as well as in humans using transcutaneous spinal stimulation.[6,87,88] However, these studies also highlight the importance of applying different timing and frequency of stimulation at the different sites.

As mentioned above, near-motor threshold stimulation amplitudes are preferable when the goal is to allow sensory information and descending input to control and modulate the motor pattern. In addition, using this approach, higher stimulation frequencies (ie, those that would lead to a rhythmic activity with high amplitudes) can be applied also for promoting a continuous (ie, nonrhythmic) motor pattern effective for standing, possibly favoring the integration of afferent and supraspinal input through the greater involvement of interneurons,[69,72] and resulting in a more physiological (ie, non pulsatile) muscle contraction.

Closed-loop spinal cord epidural stimulation
Closed-loop scES has also been tested in rats and primates for improving motor control after SCI. This approach is different than the previously described tonic, open-loop stimulation in that scES parameters are adjusted in real time, depending on kinematics or cortical feedback, with the intent to facilitate task-specific spatiotemporal patterns of motoneuron activation. For example, stimulation frequency modulation throughout the gait cycle in response to kinematics feedback optimized step height in complete rats.[89] Similarly, movement feedback was used to modulate the spatiotemporal stimulation of the spinal cord. In particular, specific "hotspots" in the dorsal roots, which targeted proprioceptive feedback circuits related to extensor or flexor muscle synergies, were stimulated depending on bilateral hindlimb kinematics feedback,

improving gait and weight bearing, among others, in SCI rats.[56] Leg motor cortex activity was also used instead of kinematics data to spatiotemporally modulate scES in a primate model, alleviating gait deficits after a thoracic unilateral corticospinal tract lesion.[90]

One of the main conceptual differences between the 2 described scES strategies seems related to the functional recovery expectations of the sensory-motor system after severe SCI. In particular, the use of tonic, nonpatterned scES to modulate the level of excitability of spinal circuits is based on the hypothesis that the human nervous system is "smart" and plastic enough to recover the ability to properly control motor pools activation based on sensory feedback and residual supraspinal input after activity-based training. On the other hand, closed-loop scES is based on the assumption that the injured sensory-motor system needs and/or would benefit from an external spatiotemporal stimulation modulation to interact with sensory information for generating optimal motoneurons activation patterns and effective movements. It will be important to understand whether the positive outcomes promoted by the closed-loop scES approach in animal models can be consistently replicated in humans with complete SCI at a chronic stage and with different neurophysiological profiles. Future studies should also clarify how closed-loop scES interacts with training-induced neural plasticity between the supraspinal and spinal centers below the level of injury.

Activity-Based Training with Spinal Cord Epidural Stimulation

Two earlier studies suggested that scES can augment training-induced plasticity, leading to improved walking in individuals with motor incomplete SCI.[91,92] The authors' research group also highlighted the importance of activity-based training with task-specific scES parameters for the progressive recovery of motor function in individuals with motor complete SCI. Training sessions involving volitional lower limb movements with scES in compete SCI individuals resulted in improved accuracy and force generation under non-weight-bearing conditions.[55] In addition, the stimulation intensity required to perform leg movements was reduced with continuous practice, suggesting positive training-induced neural adaptations between the supraspinal and spinal centers below the level of injury. The importance of training task-specificity for promoting appropriate neural plasticity was also studied in the same research participants. In particular, the authors showed that standing ability progressively improved throughout stand training with scES in all 4 individuals; however, the subsequent block of step training impaired standing in 3 out of 4 individuals.[78] This finding led the authors to ongoing studies that investigate whether different training protocols can improve the concurrent learning of standing and stepping with scES after motor complete SCI.

Long-term (∼ 3.6 years) activity-based training with scES also led to unexpected recovery of lower limb voluntary motor control and independent standing without stimulation in one of the 4 abovementioned motor complete individuals.[93] In particular, the recovery of independent standing without stimulation was observed after a 3-month training protocol that included greater training frequency (2 sessions/d), the alternated practice of standing and stepping, and an increased volitional contribution to the motor output generation. Few other human studies also showed that residual descending input to the spinal circuitry may be accessed with intense activity-based interventions to result in unexpected plasticity after chronic motor complete SCI.[6,94,95] More controlled studies on severe SCI rats also demonstrated that consistent cortical activation resulting from an active involvement during training, while the spinal cord was electrochemically modulated, was crucial for promoting neural plasticity across the lesion and related functional recovery.[96,97] Taken together, these findings suggest that (i) the human nervous system maintains remarkable recovery potential within both spinal circuitry and descending pathways after chronic motor complete SCI; (ii) the active involvement during activity-based training with scES is important even after motor complete injuries; (iii) further studies are needed to determine the optimal training "dosage" and characteristics.

FUTURE DIRECTIONS

Future studies with a larger number of SCI individuals and broader range of age and time since injury, among others, are needed to better understand the mechanisms underlying motor recovery after severe SCI using scES, as well as its potential for translation to the home and community environment. Similarly, it will be important to identify neurophysiological and imaging markers that may predict which individuals are more likely to benefit from this intervention. Technological advancements are also needed for improving flexibility and control of the stimulating device, as well as for developing training devices that can help SCI individuals to access the activity-based practice required for optimizing motor recovery.

ACKNOWLEDGMENTS

The authors thank Dr Susan Harkema for her helpful feedback on the article. The authors are supported by The Leona M. and Harry B. Helmsley Charitable Trust, Craig H. Neilsen Foundation, and Christopher & Dana Reeve Foundation.

SUPPLEMENTARY DATA

Supplementary data related to this article can be found online at https://doi.org/10.1016/j.pmr.2018.12.009.

REFERENCES

1. Harkema SJ, Schmidt-Read M, Lorenz DJ, et al. Balance and ambulation improvements in individuals with chronic incomplete spinal cord injury using locomotor training-based rehabilitation. Arch Phys Med Rehabil 2012;93(9):1508–17.
2. Jones ML, Evans N, Tefertiller C, et al. Activity-based therapy for recovery of walking in individuals with chronic spinal cord injury: results from a randomized clinical trial. Arch Phys Med Rehabil 2014;95(12):2239–46.
3. Waters RL, Yakura JS, Adkins RH, et al. Recovery following complete paraplegia. Arch Phys Med Rehabil 1992;73(9):784–9.
4. Curt A, Van Hedel HJ, Klaus D, et al. Recovery from a spinal cord injury: significance of compensation, neural plasticity, and repair. J Neurotrauma 2008; 25(6):677–85.
5. Harkema S, Gerasimenko Y, Hodes J, et al. Effect of epidural stimulation of the lumbosacral spinal cord on voluntary movement, standing, and assisted stepping after motor complete paraplegia: a case study. Lancet 2011;377(9781): 1938–47.
6. Gerasimenko YP, Lu DC, Modaber M, et al. Noninvasive reactivation of motor descending control after paralysis. J Neurotrauma 2015;32(24):1968–80.
7. Gerasimenko Y, Gorodnichev R, Machueva E, et al. Novel and direct access to the human locomotor spinal circuitry. J Neurosci 2010;30(10):3700–8.

8. Toossi A, Everaert DG, Azar A, et al. Mechanically stable intraspinal microstimulation implants for human translation. Ann Biomed Eng 2017;45(3):681–94.

9. Edgerton VR, Tillakaratne NJ, Bigbee AJ, et al. Plasticity of the spinal neural circuitry after injury. Annu Rev Neurosci 2004;27:145–67.

10. Grillner S. Neurobiological bases of rhythmic motor acts in vertebrates. Science 1985;228:143–9.

11. Harkema SJ. Plasticity of interneuronal networks of the functionally isolated human spinal cord. Brain Res Rev 2008;57(1):255–64.

12. Hubli M, Dietz V. The physiological basis of neurorehabilitation–locomotor training after spinal cord injury. J Neuroeng Rehabil 2013;10:5.

13. Hiersemenzel LP, Curt A, Dietz V. From spinal shock to spasticity: neuronal adaptations to a spinal cord injury. Neurology 2000;54(8):1574–82.

14. Beauparlant J, van den Brand R, Barraud Q, et al. Undirected compensatory plasticity contributes to neuronal dysfunction after severe spinal cord injury. Brain 2013;136(Pt 11):3347–61.

15. Dietz V. Neurophysiology of gait disorders: present and future applications. Electroencephalogr Clin Neurophysiol 1997;103(3):333–55.

16. Roy R, Harkema S, Edgerton V. Basic concepts of activity-based interventions for improved recovery of motor function after spinal cord injury. Arch Phys Med Rehabil 2012;93:1487–97.

17. Harkema SJ, Hurley SL, Patel UK, et al. Human lumbosacral spinal cord interprets loading during stepping. J Neurophysiol 1997;77(2):797–811.

18. Cote MP, Murray M, Lemay MA. Rehabilitation strategies after spinal cord injury: inquiry into the mechanisms of success and failure. J Neurotrauma 2017;34(10): 1841–57.

19. Kakulas BA. Neuropathology: the foundation for new treatments in spinal cord injury. Spinal Cord 2004;42(10):549–63.

20. McKay WB, Lim HK, Priebe MM, et al. Clinical neurophysiological assessment of residual motor control in post-spinal cord injury paralysis. Neurorehabil Neural Repair 2004;18(3):144–53.

21. Dimitrijevic MR, Dimitrijevic MM, Faganel J, et al. Suprasegmentally induced motor unit activity in paralyzed muscles of patients with established spinal cord injury. Ann Neurol 1984;16(2):216–21.

22. Sherwood AM, Dimitrijevic MR, McKay WB. Evidence of subclinical brain influence in clinically complete spinal cord injury: discomplete SCI. J Neurol Sci 1992;110(1–2):90–8.

23. Rossignol S, Martinez M, Escalona M, et al. The "beneficial" effects of locomotor training after various types of spinal lesions in cats and rats. Prog Brain Res 2015; 218:173–98.

24. De Leon RD, Hodgson JA, Roy RR, et al. Full weight-bearing hindlimb standing following stand training in the adult spinal cat. J Neurophysiol 1998;80(1):83–91.

25. de Leon RD, Hodgson JA, Roy RR, et al. Locomotor capacity attributable to step training versus spontaneous recovery after spinalization in adult cats. J Neurophysiol 1998;79(3):1329–40.

26. Edgerton VR, Roy RR. Activity-dependent plasticity of spinal locomotion: implications for sensory processing. Exerc Sport Sci Rev 2009;37(4):171–8.

27. Courtine G, Gerasimenko Y, van den BR, et al. Transformation of nonfunctional spinal circuits into functional states after the loss of brain input. Nat Neurosci 2009;12(10):1333–42.

28. Petruska JC, Ichiyama RM, Jindrich DL, et al. Changes in motoneuron properties and synaptic inputs related to step training after spinal cord transection in rats. J Neurosci 2007;27(16):4460–71.

29. Cha J, Heng C, Reinkensmeyer DJ, et al. Locomotor ability in spinal rats is dependent on the amount of activity imposed on the hindlimbs during treadmill training. J Neurotrauma 2007;24(6):1000–12.

30. Hodgson JA, Roy RR, de Leon RD, et al. Can the mammalian lumbar spinal cord learn a motor task? Med Sci Sports Exerc 1994;26(12):1491–7.

31. Bigbee AJ, Crown ED, Ferguson AR, et al. Two chronic motor training paradigms differentially influence acute instrumental learning in spinally transected rats. Behav Brain Res 2007;180(1):95–101.

32. Shah PK, Gerasimenko Y, Shyu A, et al. Variability in step training enhances locomotor recovery after a spinal cord injury. Eur J Neurosci 2012;36(1):2054–62.

33. Cai LL, Fong AJ, Otoshi CK, et al. Implications of assist-as-needed robotic step training after a complete spinal cord injury on intrinsic strategies of motor learning. J Neurosci 2006;26(41):10564–8.

34. Zewdie ET, Roy FD, Yang JF, et al. Facilitation of descending excitatory and spinal inhibitory networks from training of endurance and precision walking in participants with incomplete spinal cord injury. Prog Brain Res 2015;218:127–55.

35. Knikou M. Plasticity of corticospinal neural control after locomotor training in human spinal cord injury. Neural Plast 2012;2012:254948.

36. Sweet WH, Wepsic JG. Stimulation of the posterior columns of the spinal cord for pain control: indications, technique, and results. Clin Neurosurg 1974;21:278–310.

37. Cook AW, Weinstein SP. Chronic dorsal column stimulation in multiple sclerosis. Preliminary report. N Y State J Med 1973;73(24):2868–72.

38. Cook A. Electrical stimulation of the spinal cord. Lancet 1974;303(7862):869–70.

39. Illis LS, Oygar AE, Sedgwick EM, et al. Dorsal-column stimulation in the rehabilitation of patients with multiple sclerosis. Lancet 1976;1(7974):1383–6.

40. Waltz JM. Spinal cord stimulation: a quarter century of development and investigation. A review of its development and effectiveness in 1,336 cases. Stereotact Funct Neurosurg 1997;69(1–4 Pt 2):288–99.

41. Dooley DM, Sharkey J, Keller W, et al. Treatment of demyelinating and degenerative diseases by electro stimulation of the spinal cord. Med Prog Technol 1978;6(1):1–14.

42. Dooley DM, Sharkey J. Electrical stimulation of the spinal cord in patients with demyelinating and degenerative diseases of the central nervous system. Appl Neurophysiol 1981;44(4):218–24.

43. Siegfried J, Lazorthes Y, Broggi G. Electrical spinal cord stimulation for spastic movement disorders. Appl Neurophysiol 1981;44(1–3):77–92.

44. Richardson RR, McLone DG. Percutaneous epidural neurostimulation for paraplegic spasticity. Surg Neurol 1978;9(3):153–5.

45. Thoden U, Krainick JU, Strassburg HM, et al. Influence of dorsal column stimulation (DCS) on spastic movement disorders. Acta Neurochir (Wien) 1977;39(3–4):233–40.

46. Scerrati M, Onofrj M, Pola P. Effects of spinal cord stimulation on spasticity: H-reflex study. Appl Neurophysiol 1982;45(1–2):62–7.

47. Pinter MM, Gerstenbrand F, Dimitrijevic MR. Epidural electrical stimulation of posterior structures of the human lumbosacral cord: 3. Control of spasticity. Spinal Cord 2000;38:524–31.

48. Dimitrijevic MM, Dimitrijevic MR, Illis LS, et al. Spinal cord stimulation for the control of spasticity in patients with chronic spinal cord injury: I. Clinical observations. Cent Nerv Syst Trauma 1986;3(2):129–44.
49. Dimitrijevic MR, Illis LS, Nakajima K, et al. Spinal cord stimulation for the control of spasticity in patients with chronic spinal cord injury: II. Neurophysiologic observations. Cent Nerv Syst Trauma 1986;3(2):145–52.
50. Gaunt RA, Prochazka A, Mushahwar VK, et al. Intraspinal microstimulation excites multisegmental sensory afferents at lower stimulus levels than local alpha-motoneuron responses. J Neurophysiol 2006;96(6):2995–3005.
51. Gerasimenko YP, Lavrov IA, Courtine G, et al. Spinal cord reflexes induced by epidural spinal cord stimulation in normal awake rats. J Neurosci Methods 2006;157(2):253–63.
52. Musienko P, Heutschi J, Friedli L, et al. Multi-system neurorehabilitative strategies to restore motor functions following severe spinal cord injury. Exp Neurol 2012; 235(1):100–9.
53. Hofstoetter US, Danner SM, Freundl B, et al. Periodic modulation of repetitively elicited monosynaptic reflexes of the human lumbosacral spinal cord. J Neurophysiol 2015;114(1):400–10.
54. Danner SM, Hofstoetter US, Freundl B, et al. Human spinal locomotor control is based on flexibly organized burst generators. Brain 2015;138(Pt 3):577–88.
55. Angeli CA, Edgerton VR, Gerasimenko YP, et al. Altering spinal cord excitability enables voluntary movements after chronic complete paralysis in humans. Brain 2014;137(Pt 5):1394–409.
56. Wenger N, Moraud EM, Gandar J, et al. Spatiotemporal neuromodulation therapies engaging muscle synergies improve motor control after spinal cord injury. Nat Med 2016;22(2):138–45.
57. Moraud EM, Capogrosso M, Formento E, et al. Mechanisms underlying the neuromodulation of spinal circuits for correcting gait and balance deficits after spinal cord injury. Neuron 2016;89(4):814–28.
58. Rattay F, Minassian K, Dimitrijevic MR. Epidural electrical stimulation of posterior structures of the human lumbosacral cord: 2. quantitative analysis by computer modeling. Spinal Cord 2000;38:473–89.
59. Capogrosso M, Wenger N, Raspopovic S, et al. A computational model for epidural electrical stimulation of spinal sensorimotor circuits. J Neurosci 2013; 33(49):19326–40.
60. Arber S. Motor circuits in action: specification, connectivity, and function. Neuron 2012;74(6):975–89.
61. Ivanenko YP, Poppele RE, Lacquaniti F. Spinal cord maps of spatiotemporal alpha-motoneuron activation in humans walking at different speeds. J Neurophysiol 2006;95(2):602–18.
62. Etlin A, Blivis D, Ben-Zwi M, et al. Long and short multifunicular projections of sacral neurons are activated by sensory input to produce locomotor activity in the absence of supraspinal control. J Neurosci 2010;30(31):10324–36.
63. Nelson SG, Mendell LM. Projection of single knee flexor Ia fibers to homonymous and heteronymous motoneurons. J Neurophysiol 1978;41(3):778–87.
64. Sayenko DG, Angeli C, Harkema SJ, et al. Neuromodulation of evoked muscle potentials induced by epidural spinal-cord stimulation in paralyzed individuals. J Neurophysiol 2014;111(5):1088–99.
65. Gad P, Choe J, Nandra MS, et al. Development of a multi-electrode array for spinal cord epidural stimulation to facilitate stepping and standing after a complete spinal cord injury in adult rats. J Neuroeng Rehabil 2013;10:2.

66. Dimitrijevic MR, Gerasimenko Y, Pinter MM. Evidence for a spinal central pattern generator in humans. Ann N Y Acad Sci 1998;860(1):360–76.
67. Jilge B, Minassian K, Rattay F, et al. Initiating extension of the lower limbs in subjects with complete spinal cord injury by epidural lumbar cord stimulation. Exp Brain Res 2004;154(3):308–26.
68. Minassian K, Jilge B, Rattay F, et al. Effective spinal cord stimulation (SCS) for evoking stepping movement of paralyzed lower limbs: study of posterior root muscle reflex responses. IFESS 2002 proceedings. 2002.
69. Minassian K, Jilge B, Rattay F, et al. Stepping-like movements in humans with complete spinal cord injury induced by epidural stimulation of the lumbar cord: electromyographic study of compound muscle action potentials. Spinal Cord 2004;42(7):401–16.
70. Minassian K, Persy I, Rattay F, et al. Human lumbar cord circuitries can be activated by extrinsic tonic input to generate locomotor-like activity. Hum Mov Sci 2007;26(2):275–95.
71. Rejc E, Angeli C, Harkema S. Effects of lumbosacral spinal cord epidural stimulation for standing after chronic complete paralysis in humans. PLoS One 2015; 10(7):e0133998.
72. Jilge B, Minassian K, Rattay F, et al. Frequency-dependent selection of alternative spinal pathways with common periodic sensory input. Biol Cybern 2004;91: 359–76.
73. Altman J, Bayer SA. Development of the human spinal cord: an interpretation based on experimental studies in animals. New York: Oxford University Press; 2001.
74. Kendall FP, McCreary EK. Muscles testing and function, vol 3. Baltimore (MD): Williams & Wilkins; 1983.
75. Krames E, Peckham PH, Rezai AR. Neuromodulation: comprehensive textbook of principles, technologies, and therapies. 2nd edition. London: Academic Press is an imprint of Elsevier; 2018. ScienceDirect. Available at: https://www.sciencedirect.com/science/book/9780128053539.
76. Gerasimenko Y, Roy RR, Edgerton VR. Epidural stimulation: comparison of the spinal circuits that generate and control locomotion in rats, cats and humans. Exp Neurol 2008;209(2):417–25.
77. Murg M, Binder H, Dimitrijevic MR. Epidural electric stimulation of posterior structures of the human lumbar spinal cord: 1. Muscle twitches - a functional method to define the site of stimulation. Spinal Cord 2000;38:394–402.
78. Rejc E, Angeli CA, Bryant N, et al. Effects of stand and step training with epidural stimulation on motor function for standing in chronic complete paraplegics. J Neurotrauma 2017;34(9):1787–802.
79. Rossignol S, Dubuc R, Gossard JP. Dynamic sensorimotor interactions in locomotion. Physiol Rev 2006;86(1):89–154.
80. Musienko PE, Bogacheva IN, Gerasimenko YP. Significance of peripheral feedback in the generation of stepping movements during epidural stimulation of the spinal cord. Neurosci Behav Physiol 2007;37(2):181–90.
81. Musienko P, Courtine G, Tibbs JE, et al. Somatosensory control of balance during locomotion in decerebrated cat. J Neurophysiol 2012;107(8):2072–82.
82. Minassian K, Persy I, Rattay F, et al. Peripheral and central afferent input to the lumbar cord. Biocybern Biomed Eng 2005;25(3):11–29.
83. Grahn PJ, Lavrov IA, Sayenko DG, et al. Enabling task-specific volitional motor functions via spinal cord neuromodulation in a human with paraplegia. Mayo Clin Proc 2017;92(4):544–54.

84. Mishra AM, Pal A, Gupta D, et al. Paired motor cortex and cervical epidural electrical stimulation timed to converge in the spinal cord promotes lasting increases in motor responses. J Physiol 2017;595(22):6953–68.

85. Dose F, Deumens R, Forget P, et al. Staggered multi-site low-frequency electrostimulation effectively induces locomotor patterns in the isolated rat spinal cord. Spinal Cord 2016;54(2):93–101.

86. Shah PK, Sureddi S, Alam M, et al. Unique spatiotemporal neuromodulation of the lumbosacral circuitry shapes locomotor success after spinal cord injury. J Neurotrauma 2016;33(18):1709–23.

87. Gerasimenko Y, Gorodnichev R, Moshonkina T, et al. Transcutaneous electrical spinal-cord stimulation in humans. Ann Phys Rehabil Med 2015;58(4):225–31.

88. Gerasimenko Y, Gad P, Sayenko D, et al. Integration of sensory, spinal, and volitional descending inputs in regulation of human locomotion. J Neurophysiol 2016; 116(1):98–105.

89. Wenger N, Moraud EM, Raspopovic S, et al. Closed-loop neuromodulation of spinal sensorimotor circuits controls refined locomotion after complete spinal cord injury. Sci Transl Med 2014;6(255):255ra133.

90. Capogrosso M, Milekovic T, Borton D, et al. A brain–spine interface alleviating gait deficits after spinal cord injury in primates. Nature 2016;539(7628):284–8.

91. Herman R, He J, D'Luzansky S, et al. Spinal cord stimulation facilitates functional walking in a chronic, incomplete spinal cord injured. Spinal Cord 2002;40(2): 65–8.

92. Carhart MR, He J, Herman R, et al. Epidural spinal-cord stimulation facilitates recovery of functional walking following incomplete spinal-cord injury. IEEE Trans Neural Syst Rehabil Eng 2004;12(1):32–42.

93. Rejc E, Angeli CA, Atkinson D, et al. Motor recovery after activity-based training with spinal cord epidural stimulation in a chronic motor complete paraplegic. Sci Rep 2017;7(1):13476.

94. Donati AR, Shokur S, Morya E, et al. Long-term training with a brain-machine interface-based gait protocol induces partial neurological recovery in paraplegic patients. Sci Rep 2016;6:30383.

95. Possover M. Recovery of sensory and supraspinal control of leg movement in people with chronic paraplegia: a case series. Arch Phys Med Rehabil 2014; 95(4):610–4.

96. Asboth L, Friedli L, Beauparlant J, et al. Cortico-reticulo-spinal circuit reorganization enables functional recovery after severe spinal cord contusion. Nat Neurosci 2018;21(4):576–88.

97. van den Brand R, Heutschi J, Barraud Q, et al. Restoring voluntary control of locomotion after paralyzing spinal cord injury. Science 2012;336(6085):1182–5.

Gait Segmentation of Data Collected by Instrumented Shoes Using a Recurrent Neural Network Classifier

Antonio Prado, BS, MSc[a], Xiya Cao, BS[a],
Maxime T. Robert, MSc, PhD[b], Andrew M. Gordon, PhD[b],
Sunil K. Agrawal, MSc, PhD[c],*

KEYWORDS

- Wearables • Gait recognition • Machine learning • Neural network
- Rehabilitation robotics

KEY POINTS

- Recurrent Neural Networks and instrumented footwear can be combined to generate reliable gait characteristics in near real time.
- DeepSole is a portable system for gait characterization, is designed to be unobtrusive to the user, and can be used outside a clinic setting.
- The Neural Network model can be used to segment gait information without needing specific calibration.

INTRODUCTION

Gait analysis allows clinicians and researchers to quantitatively characterize the kinematics and kinetics of human movement. Sensor-based gait characterization systems are recognized as clinical tools to analyze patient mobility.[1] For example, quantitative gait data have been used to determine the need for surgery in children with cerebral palsy (CP) and to prescribe the care and treatment after surgery.[2] Furthermore, Wren and colleagues[3] showed that children with CP who underwent clinical gait analysis before lower extremity orthopedic surgery had significantly lower incidence of additional surgery.

Disclosure Statement: The authors have nothing to disclose.
[a] Mechanical Engineering, Columbia University, 500 West 120th Street, New York, NY 10027, USA; [b] Department of Biobehavioral Sciences, Teachers College, Columbia University, 525 West 120th Street, Box 93, New York, NY 10027, USA; [c] Columbia University, 500 West 120th Street, Mail Code: 4703, New York, NY 10027, USA
* Corresponding author.
E-mail address: sunil.agrawal@columbia.edu

Phys Med Rehabil Clin N Am 30 (2019) 355–366
https://doi.org/10.1016/j.pmr.2018.12.007
1047-9651/19/© 2018 Elsevier Inc. All rights reserved.

Devices that quantify gait can be either portable, such as instrumented shoes, or nonportable, such as motion capture systems and instrumented walkways. There is a tradeoff between these 2 classes of systems in terms of portability and accuracy. However, recent computer advances allow for the collection of meaningful data outside of the clinical setting, over different terrains, and activities.[4] These devices are critical for recording abnormal walking behaviors, for example, episodic phenomena like freezing of gait of patients with Parkinson disease.[5] Although the portable devices permit longer recordings in natural environments, the added flexibility increases the potential for sensor misinterpretation. This error can be significant when used on participants with irregular walking, such as the elderly, or individuals with CP, adding to the complexity of data processing.

Gait characterization typically includes both spatial and temporal parameters. These parameters can quantify changes in the user locomotion and can track progress of training or rehabilitation. For example, stride to stride fluctuations can be used to assess risk of falls,[6,7] and gait variability has been used as a good predictor for dementia.[8,9]

To analyze the collected data, most techniques involve 2 stages: (i) segmenting the data into steps or strides to calculate temporal parameters, and then, (ii) estimating the spatial parameters using the segmented data. The initial contact time, usually made by the heel, is set as the start of the gait cycle.[10] Different algorithms have been proposed to obtain gait characteristics, from simple thresholding algorithms[11] to machine learning algorithms.[12,13] These methods analyze the sensor readings but require human effort to validate and "clean" the data, for example, for removing sensor errors or noise. This step is a time-intensive step and prone to errors because only a limited number of features during the sensor measurements can be considered, for example, pressure or inertial measurements. The methods mentioned above provide good performance but rely on the skills of a person analyzing the data to find the important features in the recorded gait. Also, algorithms need to be formulated to identify these engineered features. The difficulty of finding these features increases as the number of sensors grows. However, limiting the number and types of sensors introduces the risk that data cannot be processed if the device malfunctions.

A model specifically created to reliably identify and characterize a person's gait using the raw data, without any preprocessing, would greatly reduced the time needed to obtain meaningful data. The model would allow researchers and clinicians to record and analyze long walking sessions outside the clinical environment. However, it is critical to maintain equivalent accuracy and precision when compared with the state-of-the-art methods, while still significantly reducing the processing time.

Machine learning allows automation of tedious processes and greatly reduces the time needed to obtain meaningful output data. Hannink and colleagues[14] used Convolution Neural Networks to obtain spatiotemporal gait parameters from an inertial sensor with performance comparable to state-of-the-art devices. Mannini and Sabatini[12] created a gait segmentation algorithm using Hidden Markov Models with signals acquired from a gyroscope mounted at the foot. They obtained an accuracy of 98.3% when considering an event identified by a rejection window less than ± 30 milliseconds. For their experiment, they used only 3 healthy participants walking on a treadmill for 2 minutes at various speeds and inclines.

López-Nava and colleagues[13] used a Bayesian model to estimate the temporal gait parameters of 10 healthy participants over three 7.6-m laps at a comfortable walking speed. Only the acceleration data were recorded and processed, showing accuracy and precision (absolute error $\pm$ standard deviation) of 9.1 ± 6.5 milliseconds for step time, 42.3 ± 20.2 milliseconds for stance phase time, and 32.2 ± 13.9 milliseconds for swing time.

Artificial Neural Networks (ANN) allow the mapping of an input vector X to an output vector Y, where the input and output can be multidimensional.[15] The algorithm looks at a single event through different sensors and merges this information in their mapping, thus avoiding the need to manually program algorithms that recognize engineered features. For time-series data, the ANN commonly used are either Convolutional Neural Networks (CNN) or Recurrent Neural Networks (RNN). CNN are specialized for processing data that have a gridlike topology[16] and have been successfully used to identify human motion from the signal of several Inertial Measurement Units (IMU).[17] RNN are models with the ability to sequentially process information one element at a time, generating a sequence-to-sequence mapping.[18] They excel at determining outputs from inputs that are not independent.[19] RNN are more desirable than CNN because they accumulate data, capturing long-range time dependencies.[19]

This article presents an RNN model that classifies the recordings from an instrumented shoe. The model output is used to segment the walking data and to calculate temporal characteristics of the gait. RNN was chosen over CNN because it provides an output for every intermediate step of the network.[15] This model property was used to reduce the number of incorrect predictions. The input to the network is the data of 3 pressure sensors, a 3-axis accelerometer, and Euler angles of the feet. Here, the authors show that using the RNN classifier, they can segment the walking data within seconds without human intervention.

PARTICIPANTS

The data set used for the training and evaluation of the model consists of 28 healthy participants greater than 18 years old (8 women and 20 men, aged 19–31). A second data set of 7 children (4 girls and 3 boys, aged 7–14) with CP was collected and used for evaluation. Participant characteristics are listed in **Tables 1** and **2**. For the CP group, the Manual Ability Classification System (MACS) and Gross Motor Function Classification System (GMFCS), affected side, and lesion type are reported. Because the experiment of walking with shoes is noninvasive, the only requirement to participate in the experiment was the ability to walk independently for 6 minutes. None of the participants used assistive devices during their testing.

For the CP group, the inclusion criteria were that they were diagnosed with unilateral CP, that they were able to walk for 6 minutes without any assistance, that they were cooperative, and that they were aged between 6 and 17 years old. People who presented with other neurologic disorders, for example, orthopedic surgery or botulinum toxin injections, on the affected leg within 6 months were excluded from the experiment.

Table 1
Participant characteristics for cerebral palsy group

ID	Height (cm)	Weight (kg)	Shoe	Gender	Age	Affected Side	MACS	GMFCS	Lesion Type
CP001	185	94	12	M	15	Left	II	I	MCA
CP002	170	52	12	M	14	Left	II	I	PVL
CP003	132	24	6	W	10	Left	II	II	PVL
CP004	152	52	6	W	12	Right	I	I	MCA
CP005	137	42	5	W	8	Left	III	II	PVL
CP006	138	27	5	W	9	Left	III	II	PVL
CP007	155	33	7	M	14	Left	II	I	PVL

Table 2
Results by group and event in milliseconds

	NIT		IT		CP	
Event	ME ± SD	MAE ± SD	ME ± SD	MAE ± SD	ME ± SD	MAE ± SD
HS	−5.9 ± 37.1	23.9 ± 29.0	−8.3 ± 23.5	16.8 ± 18.5	26.4 ± 46.0	35.2 ± 39.7
TO	11.4 ± 47.4	35.9 ± 32.8	10.7 ± 42.3	32.8 ± 28.7	21.0 ± 94.6	68.6 ± 68.6

DeepSole SYSTEM

DeepSole is the next iteration of the modular instrumented footwear developed at Columbia University Robotics and Rehabilitation Laboratory. The earlier version, called SoleSound, was presented by Minto and colleagues.[20] This new version has several improvements in order to make it more portable, reliable, and durable. The system consists of 2 foot modules, each with a pressure-sensitive insole, 3 vibration motors, a 9 Degree of Freedom (DoF) IMU, and a microcontroller (**Fig. 1**). The microcontrollers sample the sensors at 200 Hz, record the data to a MicroSD card, and stream it over UDP for real-time visualization.

Each insole consists of 3 pressure areas: one located under the phalanges, the second located under the metatarsals, and the third located under the calcaneus. The pressure sensors are made with a layer of piezoresistive fabric (Eontex, CA, USA) in between 2 layers of conductive copper fabric. These sensors can be custom made to any shape and retain their piezoresistive properties. They provide an average loading of each independent area instead of just a single point. This feature is especially useful when characterizing populations with irregular loading during gait, such as children with CP. The vibration motors are located under the first and fifth metatarsals, and the calcaneus. Each can be controlled independently to change the vibration intensity. The system can be donned in minutes and is similar to putting on a regular pair of shoes. Because of the soft materials used, the insoles are indistinguishable by the wearer.

CLINICAL TESTING

The participants were asked to perform the 6-minute walk test[21] while wearing the DeepSole system. During this test, a subject walked at a self-selected speed for 6 minutes in a hallway equipped with a Zeno Walkway (Protokinetics, PA, USA). The

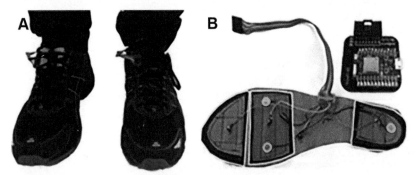

Fig. 1. (*A*) Subject wearing the DeepSole system. (*B*) Printed circuit board with microcontroller and IMU, and instrumented insole with pressure sensors (*yellow outline*) and vibration motors (*green outline*).

walkway has a total length of 6 meters, but 2 meters were added to the extremes of the walkway to make a total walking distance of 10 meters. Data were recorded simultaneously from both systems. Parents and children signed informed consent/child-assent forms approved by the Columbia University Medical Center Ethics Committee.

METHODS

Segmentation is the step of gait analysis that involves splitting the data into cycles. Each cycle is defined by Heel Strikes (HS) and Toe Offs (TO). Even though several algorithms exist to identify these events, they usually involve supervision and intervention from a human to identify faulty cycles. False positives can come either from sensor errors or from gait variability of the participants. Identifying faulty cycles is time intensive and could take the user between 1 hour and 12+ hours to analyze 6 minutes of walking data of each subject.

Using HS and TO, the authors can segment data and calculate 15+ spatial gait parameters. A graphical example of the different gait events and how to identify these using only HS and TO events is shown in **Fig. 2**. With the authors' proposed algorithm, they wish to substitute commonly used thresholding algorithm to segment the data. The thresholding algorithms are ineffective when the user has an abnormal gait, because the pressure data can be erratic and a single threshold value may not be sufficient for the entire recording.

NEURAL NETWORKS

The recordings were resampled from 200 Hz to 100 Hz to reduce the high-frequency noise and the computational load. After this down-sampling, no other preprocessing was done except for appending the readings to create a matrix.

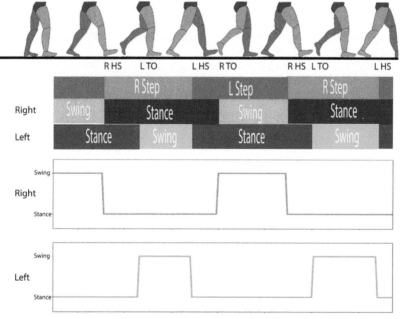

Fig. 2. (*Top*) Normal gait cycle and how the events are defined by HS and TO. (*Bottom*) An example of a binary function of the gait phases.

From the DeepSole, the authors obtained 9 signals: 3 pressure sensor readings, 3 linear accelerations, and 3 Euler angles. The last 20 readings from the sensors are appended into a matrix $X \varepsilon R^{20 \times 9}$ to use as inputs to the RNN. Here, the columns represented the values of the signals, and the rows represent the time when the signals were recorded. The last row is the current reading at time (t) and first row is the readings at time ($t-19 * d_t$), where d_t is the sampling time of 10 milliseconds. In the training set, the left- and right-side recordings were used indiscriminately. This training strategy allowed the model to classify the data using information only from the desired side. Using only the desired side makes the model suitable for predicting symmetric and asymmetric gait, because each side is predicted independently.

Because HS and TO are very short time events, creating a model to identify these events would be impractical. Therefore, the gait cycle was split into the phases of a step, and the HS and TO information was later reconstructed from this output. Using this approach, several training samples can be obtained from a single step instead of only 2 per step, one for HS and one for TO. The Network is an RNN classifier with 2 classes: stance phase and swing phase. Using this strategy, the model can generate a function of time showing the phase of the gait. By using the differentiation of the output, one can identify HS as going from off the ground to on the ground ($\dot{y} = -1$), and TO as the point where the foot is no longer in contact with the ground ($\dot{y} = 1$).

The output of the network is a binary function of time that shows the phases of the gait:

$$y(t) = \begin{cases} 0 & \textit{Stance Phase} \\ 1 & \textit{Swing Phase} \end{cases} \qquad (1)$$

Fig. 3 shows a schematic of the model's architecture. First, the input matrix is normalized per channel and is fed into an RNN containing 8 layers, each with 20 Gated Recurrent Unit (GRU) cells.[22]

From the RNN, a matrix $R \varepsilon R^{20 \times 20}$ is obtained, where every row i corresponds to the predicted value of $y(i + 1)$, and $i = 20$ is equivalent to the current time t.[18] This matrix is used in the classification layers.

At this point, the model splits into 2 outputs: one part gives the expected values for $y(t)$ to ($t - 10$) using rows $i = 9$ to $i = 19$ from matrix R and the following equations:

$$j = 19 - n \qquad (2)$$

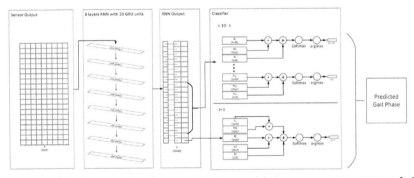

Fig. 3. Network Architecture for the segmentation model. Sensor measurements are fed to an RNN with GRU units; the output is then passed through a classifier to obtain the prediction for $t + 1$.

$$y(t - n) = \text{argmax}\left(\text{softmax}\left(R_j W_j + b_j\right)\right) \tag{3}$$

where $y(t - n)$ is the predicted value at time $t - n$, R_j is the jth row of matrix R, $W_j \varepsilon \mathbb{R}^{20 \times 2}$ is a weight matrix, and $b_j \varepsilon \mathbb{R}^{1 \times 2}$ is a bias vector.

The second output predicts the value of $y(t + 1)$ by considering the previous values of y using

$$y(t+1) = \text{argmax}\left(\text{softmax}\left(R_t W_t + y_p W_p + b_t\right)\right) \tag{4}$$

$$y_p = \begin{cases} y_{true} & \text{if training} \\ y_{predicted} & \text{if evaluation} \end{cases} \tag{5}$$

where $y(t + 1)$ is the predicted time for the next location of the foot given the past 20 sensor readings, R_t is the last row of matrix R, $W_t \varepsilon \mathbb{R}^{20 \times 2}$, $W_p \varepsilon \mathbb{R}^{10 \times 2}$ are weight matrices, and $b_t \varepsilon \mathbb{R}^{1 \times 2}$ is a bias vector. y_p is a row vector containing the last 10 values of the output $y(t)$. During training, these values are fed from the training set, but during run and evaluation the predictions obtained from equation 3 are used.

In equations 3 and 4, the *softmax* activation and the *argmax* combined to create a "1-of-2" encoding, winner-takes-all of the outputs.[23] The *softmax* function is used to represent the probability distribution over 2 classes,[16] and *argmax* is used to choose the class with the highest probability.

Each model was trained for 200 epochs, that is, the model goes 200 times through the data set using an Adams optimizer[24] to minimize the cross-entropy loss function (6).

$$H_{y'}(y) = -\sum_i y'_i \log(y_i)$$

Google TensorFlow library[25] was used to implement and train the network.

EVALUATION

The model presented is a classifier of the gait phase, that is, 0 for stance and 1 for swing. To obtain meaningful gait characteristics, one must identify the HS and the TO events.

Given the model architecture, at every time t, 2 outputs are provided, the predicted phase and the expected phase for the last 10 measurements, which means that after 10 system cycles, at every time t, there are 10 values for the position of the foot at time t. By rounding the mean of all 10 predictions, the output can reduce the number of false predictions. The reduction is particularly useful at the HS and TO gait events, because these are located at the transition between states and should be singleton events per step cycle.

To test the performance of the algorithm, a "leave-one-out cross-validation" (LOOCV) test was performed over the P participants ($P = 28$). A total of P models were trained with $P - 1$ participants.[26] The LOOCV was repeated P times excluding a different subject for every iteration. For each of the P models created, the dimensions of the training data sets were kept constant by randomly selecting 5000 samples from each subject (2500 stance phase and 2500 swing phase samples). Using 5000 samples per subject means that for training, only 50 seconds out of the 6 minutes recorded were used. By decoupling the effects of the participants involved in the training, this cross-validation allows performance evaluation of the learning ability of the network architecture.

Two participants were selected and tested with each model (28 total for each group). The participants were divided into 2 categories: In-Training (IT) and Not-In-Training (NIT). NIT members are the participants left out of the training for the model tested. IT were participants, picked at random, whose step information were used during the training of a particular model. Each subject was tested 2 times, once as part of IT and once as part of NIT. If the classification performance of the network and error ranges is similar between groups, the model could be used with unknown participants without the need for a calibration session.

The model with the highest test accuracy was used with a data set of 7 children with CP. To assess the performance of the RNN, the HS and TO identified were compared against the walkway recording. Each event was paired using a maximum search window of 0.5 seconds to identify the corresponding step. Each event required the HS and TO to be identified. If any was missing, the event was counted as unidentified and was not used for the error calculation. The mean errors (ME) and mean absolute errors (MAE) were used to quantify the accuracy and precision of the RNN.

RESULTS

During the training, the 28 models achieved a mean accuracy (ME $\pm$ SD) for classifying the gait phase (equation 1) of 91.45% $\pm$ 0.27% for y at time $t + 1$ (equation 4), and 91.03% $\pm$ 0.21% for y_p (equation 3) at time $t - 9$ to time t on the training data set. For the test data set, the mean accuracy was 89.20% $\pm$ 4.73% for $y(t + 1)$ and 89.08% $\pm$ 4.64% for y_p.

The model was able to identify 4138 out of 4198 steps for NIT comparison, each step an HS and TO, for 28 participants over 6 minutes of walking; this is a 98.6% identification rate. For the IT group, it identified 99.4% of the steps (4174). For the CP group, the RNN identified 1776 out of 2192 steps for the 7 participants; this is an 81.0% rate.

For the NIT group, the model was able to achieve an accuracy and precision (ME $\pm$ SD) of -5.9 ± 37.1 milliseconds for HS and 11.4 ± 47.4 milliseconds for TO. The IT group achieved an accuracy and precision of -8.3 ± 23.5 milliseconds for HS and 10.7 ± 42.3 milliseconds for TO. For the CP group, the model achieved 26.4 ± 46.0 milliseconds for HS and 21.0 ± 94.6 milliseconds for TO. Results showing the ME and the Root Mean Square Error (RMSE) are presented in **Table 1** for both healthy groups tested and for the CP group.

The error histogram and the Bland-Altman plots[27] between the RNN and the reference system for the 3 groups and the 2 events are presented in **Figs. 4** and **5**. The Bland-Altman plots show that the performance of the Neural Network (NN) is maintained over the complete recording.

DISCUSSION

The algorithm was tested with a data set of 28 adult participants and 7 children with CP. The model was able to use the full range of sensors to segment the data even when sensor error was present (**Fig. 6**). The classification capabilities were maintained when the subject was not involved in the training. The classification was tested using LOOCV; the precision and accuracy were maintained between the NIT and IT groups. The similar performance between groups shows that the RNN architecture learned to classify the gait by using the multidimensional space created by the pressure and inertial sensors and could be used without subject-specific calibration.

The results in this study show that the algorithm presented, based on RNN for segmentation and estimation of temporal parameters of gait, provides reliable

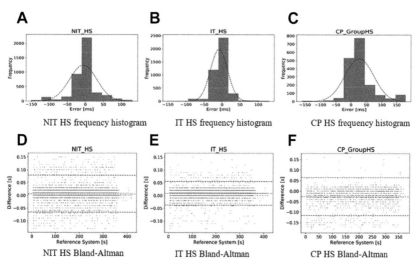

Fig. 4. Error distributions of the identification errors for HS with respect to the reference system. (*A–C*) Histogram of the error distributions for the 3 groups. (*D–F*) The Band-Altman plots show the bounding error for HS for the NIT, IT, and CP groups.

performance compared with a commonly used instrumented walkway when tested with healthy adults. Furthermore, it has a similar accuracy and performance to other Machine Learning algorithms that use techniques like Hidden Markov Models or Bayesian Models, even when it was tested with more than 200 minutes of walking.

Even though the RNN had a diminished accuracy and identification rate when used with children with CP, the results are encouraging, especially when it is considered

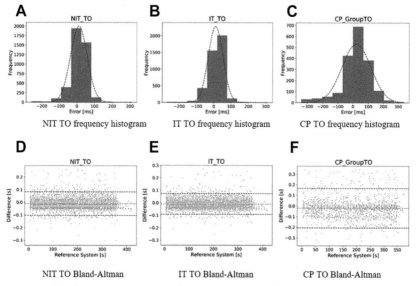

Fig. 5. Error distributions of the identification errors for TO with respect to the reference system. (*A–C*) Histogram of the error distributions for the 3 groups. (*D–F*) The Bland-Altman plots show the bounding error for TO for the NIT, IT, and CP groups.

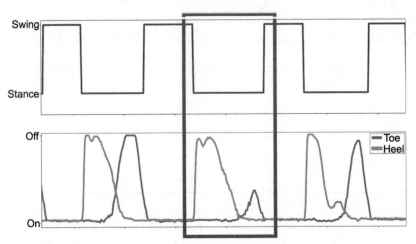

Fig. 6. Sensor error due to variability in the walking characteristics of subjects. RNN Model can classify the data despite the misreading. Only Heel (calcaneus) and Toe (distal phalanx) are shown for clarity.

that the RNN was trained with young adults and it had never seen data from children, let alone those with CP. As shown by Wren and colleagues,[28] children with CP often present with gait abnormalities, such as equinus and calcaneus, and in-toeing and out-toeing. The abnormalities make processing the recordings even with a reference system challenging and time consuming, because it involves manual correction. With the RNN, the processing of all 7 participants took only seconds. The fast processing speed means that the algorithm may be used with long recordings outside of a clinic environment, where even an 80% detection rate can still provide the overall trends of the gait. Also, the authors think that by increasing the number of participants with CP and combining the data sets between adult and children participants, models can be created that are usable on both populations.

SUMMARY

The proposed model architecture uses the parallel nature of the neural network toolboxes and its ability to compile the model for fast execution. The processing time for the complete data set, without any preprocessing to clean the data, was reduced from hours per subject to less than 1 second. This time performance boost and the portability of the instrumented shoes open the possibility to record longer sessions outside clinical settings.

With the hardware used, one could classify the gait events in real time, at a frequency of 10 to 20 Hz. It has been shown that during walking, most frequencies of human movement are less than 6 Hz.[10] Thus, this processing speed would be enough to capture the kinematics and kinetics during walking. By using the properties of sequence-to-sequence mapping from raw sensor data to abstract motion characteristics, ANN could be used as a real-time sensor for human motion. This sensor could be used by other devices, like exoskeletons, or those that provide feedback during episodic events, such as Freezing of Gait in Parkinson disease.[29] In the near future, the authors plan to test the NN to obtain spatial parameters as well as temporal parameters. All these advances would remove setting and time restrictions on gait analysis.

ACKNOWLEDGMENTS

The first author of this article was partially supported by the Mexican National Council for Science and Technology (CONACYT). M.T.R. was supported by a postdoctoral training award from Fonds de Recherche en Sante du Quebec.

REFERENCES

1. Simon SR. Quantification of human motion: gait analysis—benefits and limitations to its application to clinical problems. J Biomech 2004;37(12):1869–80.
2. Kay RM, Dennis S, Rethlefsen S, et al. The effect of preoperative gait analysis on orthopaedic decision making. Clin Orthop Relat Res 2000;372:217–22.
3. Wren TAL, Kalisvaart MM, Ghatan CE, et al. Effects of preoperative gait analysis on costs and amount of surgery. J Pediatr Orthop 2009;29(6):558–63.
4. Xu W, Huang M-C, Amini N, et al. Smart insole: a wearable system for gait analysis. In: Proceedings of the 5th International Conference on PErvasive Technologies Related to assistive environments. New York: ACM Press; 2012. p. 18.
5. Winfree KN, Pretzer-Aboff I, Hilgart D, et al. The effect of step-synchronized vibration on patients with Parkinson's disease: case studies on subjects with freezing of gait or an implanted deep brain stimulator. IEEE Trans Neural Syst Rehabil Eng 2013;21(5):806–11.
6. Hausdorff JM. Gait dynamics, fractals and falls: finding meaning in the stride-to-stride fluctuations of human walking. Hum Mov Sci 2007;26(4):555–89.
7. Maki BE. Gait changes in older adults: predictors of falls or indicators of fear? J Am Geriatr Soc 1997;45(3):313–20.
8. Verghese J, Lipton RB, Hall CB, et al. Abnormality of gait as a predictor of non-Alzheimer's dementia. N Engl J Med 2002;347(22):1761–8.
9. Buracchio T, Dodge HH, Howieson D, et al. The trajectory of gait speed preceding mild cognitive impairment. Arch Neurol 2010;67(8):980–6.
10. Winter DA. Biomechanics and motor control of human movement. John Wiley & Sons; 2009.
11. Hausdorff JM, Ladin Z, Wei JY. Footswitch system for measurement of the temporal parameters of gait. J Biomech 1995;28(3):347–51.
12. Mannini A, Sabatini AM. A hidden Markov model-based technique for gait segmentation using a foot-mounted gyroscope. In: 2011 Annual International Conference of the IEEE Engineering in Medicine and Biology Society, EMBC. IEEE. 2011:4369–73. doi:10.1109/IEMBS.2011.6091084.
13. López-Nava IH, Muñoz-Meléndez A, Pérez Sanpablo AI, et al. Estimation of temporal gait parameters using Bayesian models on acceleration signals. Comput Methods Biomech Biomed Engin 2016;19(4):396–403.
14. Hannink J, Kautz T, Pasluosta CF, et al. Sensor-based gait parameter extraction with deep convolutional neural networks. IEEE J Biomed Health Inform 2017; 21(1):85–93.
15. Graves A. Supervised sequence labelling with recurrent neural networks. Springer; 2012.
16. Goodfellow I, Bengio Y, Courville A. Deep learning. MIT Press; 2016.
17. Yang JB, Nguyen MN, San PP, et al. Deep convolutional neural networks on multi-channel time series for human activity recognition. In Ijcai, Vol. 15. p. 3995–4001.
18. Sutskever I, Vinyals O, Le QV. Sequence to sequence learning with neural networks 2014. In Advances in neural information processing systems, p. 3104–12.

19. Lipton ZC, Berkowitz J, Elkan C. A critical review of recurrent neural networks for sequence learning 2015. Available at: http://arxiv.org/abs/1506.00019. Accessed October 1, 2017.
20. Minto S, Zanotto D, Boggs EM, et al. Validation of a footwear-based gait analysis system with action-related feedback. IEEE Trans Neural Syst Rehabil Eng 2016; 24(9):971–80.
21. ATS Committee on Proficiency Standards for Clinical Pulmonary Function Laboratories. ATS statement: guidelines for the six-minute walk test. Am J Respir Crit Care Med 2002;166(1):111–7.
22. Cho K, van Merrienboer B, Gulcehre C, et al. Learning phrase representations using RNN encoder-decoder for statistical machine translation. 2014. Available at: http://arxiv.org/abs/1406.1078. Accessed October 1, 2017.
23. Hüsken M, Stagge P. Recurrent neural networks for time series classification. Neurocomputing 2003;50:223–35.
24. Kingma DP, Ba J. Adam: a method for stochastic optimization. 2014. Available at: http://arxiv.org/abs/1412.6980. Accessed September 25, 2017.
25. Abadi M, Barham, P, Chen J, et al. Tensorflow: a system for large-scale machine learning. In OSDI. 2016; Vol 16. p. 265–83.
26. Duda RO, Hart PE, Stork DG. Pattern classification. International Journal of Computational Intelligence and Applications 2001;1:335–9.
27. Bland JM, Altman DG. Statistical methods for assessing agreement between two methods of clinical measurement. The lancet 1986;327(8476):307–10.
28. Wren TAL, Rethlefsen S, Kay RM. Prevalence of specific gait abnormalities in children with cerebral palsy: Influence of cerebral palsy subtype, age, and previous surgery. J Pediatr Orthop 2005;25(1):79–83.
29. Mazilu S, Blanke U, Hardegger M, et al. GaitAssist: a daily-life support and training system for parkinson's disease patients with freezing of gait. In Proceedings of the 32nd annual ACM conference on Human factors in computing systems. New York: ACM Press; 2014:2531–40.

Robot-assisted Therapy for the Upper Limb after Cervical Spinal Cord Injury

Nuray Yozbatiran, PT, PhD[a],*, Gerard E. Francisco, MD[b]

KEYWORDS

• Spinal cord injury • Robotic-assisted training • Upper limb • Functional recovery

KEY POINTS

• Tetraplegia, resulting from cervical injury is the most frequent neurologic category after spinal cord injury and causes substantial disability.
• Improving arm and hand functions after cervical spinal cord injury is a major determinant of independence and life quality.
• Robotic devices hold promise to deliver high-intensity, repetitive, adaptive training.
• Robot-assisted rehabilitation of upper limb after cervical spinal cord injury is safe and feasible but lacks sufficient evidence of clinical effectiveness.

INTRODUCTION

Spinal Cord Injury Facts and Figures with a Specific Focus on Tetraplegia

Spinal cord injury (SCI) is considered one of the most devastating injuries that causes lifelong disability. Each year approximately 17,700 people suffer from SCI in the United States, and approximately 47% of these affect the cervical spine, causing mild to severe impairment in arm and hand functions.[1] SCI affects primarily young adults, with an average age at injury of 41 years and average lifetime costs exceeding $1 million per person in the United States. Although more than half of persons with SCI reported being employed at the time of injury, only 12% are employed 1 year after injury. Tetraplegia from cervical injury is the most common neurologic category of SCI.[2] Depending on the type (complete vs incomplete) and level of injury (cervical vertebrae

The authors have nothing to disclose.
[a] Department of Physical Medicine and Rehabilitation, McGovern Medical School, The University of Texas Health Science Center at Houston, NeuroRecovery Research Center at TIRR Memorial Hermann, 1333 Moursund Street, Room 315, Houston, TX 77030, USA; [b] Department of Physical Medicine and Rehabilitation, McGovern Medical School, The University of Texas Health Science Center at Houston, NeuroRecovery Research Center at TIRR Memorial Hermann, 1333 Moursund Street, Suite E-108, Houston, TX 77030, USA
* Corresponding author.
E-mail address: Nuray.Yozbatiran@uth.tmc.edu

Phys Med Rehabil Clin N Am 30 (2019) 367–384
https://doi.org/10.1016/j.pmr.2018.12.008
1047-9651/19/© 2018 Elsevier Inc. All rights reserved.

C4–C7), the level of assistance each individual requires ranges from complete caregiver-dependent to partially functional in activities of daily living, social and recreational activities, and work-related activities.

Given that a majority of SCI individuals are in their most productive years, with a life expectancy approaching those of the healthy population, more aggressive treatment strategies focusing on improvement of peripheral muscle control as well as recovery of central nervous system (CNS) are needed.

Arm and hand functions are among the major determinants of independence in daily activities, such as self-care, feeding, toilet transfers, chair or wheelchair transfers, tub transfers, and bed mobility, and in social and work-related activities. After cervical SCI, affected individuals experience substantial or complete loss of arm and hand function.[3] In several studies, more than half of people with tetraplegia reported that regaining arm and hand functions would most improve their quality of life.[4,5]

The residual strength of partially paralyzed muscles is an important determinant of independence and function in tetraplegia. Therefore, small improvements in upper extremity function can make a clinically significant difference in feeding, bathing, transfer, and other functional activities.[6] For example, the strength of the wrist extensor muscles has a significant impact on hand function in people with C6 injuries (tenodesis effect).

Rehabilitation After Cervical Spinal Cord Injury

Since the work by Santiago Ramon y Cajal in 1928,[7] the common assumption has been that the CNS is hard-wired, which means incapable of modification anatomically and incapable of repairing itself. To some extent this assumption might have affected the approach of rehabilitation specialists in designing treatment protocols so that education in compensatory techniques to regain independence in daily activities, such as using assistive devices to accomplish eating, dressing, and transfers, has been emphasized over treatments to facilitate neural recovery. Over the past 3 decades, however, this view of the CNS has undergone fundamental change. Numerous studies from basic science provide evidence that the brain is capable of producing new functional nerve cells and that these neurons are interconnected with existing nerve cells. Even more important, however, is that after injury or in the course of neurodegenerative diseases, the brain and spinal cord have the ability to reorganize synaptic connections.[8,9] Therefore, understanding brain and spinal cord plasticity provides a basis for developing better treatment interventions to facilitate return of functions after injury.

There have been multiple efforts to translate evidence from animal studies into clinical practice to promote recovery of motor function in humans. One example of this type of plasticity is studies where cats with complete spinal transections respond to intense walking training in the absence of supraspinal input. Most research on exercise training post-SCI has been done in gait training whereas studies on motor recovery of arm and hand functions after SCI are limited and generally focus on peripheral muscle control rather than neurorecovery per se. For example, functional electrical stimulation[10] exercise, biofeedback, and botulinum toxin injections[11] are aimed at sensory-motor recovery; neuroprostheses,[12] and brain-computer interface systems[13] increase motor control through alternative communication and control systems; surgical interventions, such as tendon transfers, offer permanent changes to muscle structure.[14]

Activity-based intervention in SCI rehabilitation provides facilitation to the CNS through intense, repetitive, and rhythmic activities. More clinical trials are needed to promote recovery of upper limb movements within the context of facilitating neural networks at the spinal and supraspinal levels, thereby inducing intrinsic recovery mechanism and improving functions.

Robot-assisted Upper Limb Rehabilitation

Optimization of treatment protocols should focus not only on questions, such as context and when, but also on how much.[15] Recent work in neuroscience demonstrates that treatment intensity has important effects on motor recovery, and, even years after a neurologic injury, neuroplasticity of the adult brain can be impacted by experience (activity-based therapy). Robotic-assisted therapy, in addition to traditional therapy, has potential to support recovery by delivering high-intensity motor practices.[16–19]

In the past decade, introduction of robotic devices into rehabilitation has enabled semiautomated or automated high-intensity repetitive therapy, which otherwise would be quite labor intensive.[20–22] Although the extent of preservation of spinal tracts is an important determinant of residual motor function, neuronal circuits below the level of lesion can be activated by appropriate afferent input, even in the absence of supraspinal input.[23] For example, in recovery of locomotor functions, 10% to 15% of intact descending spinal tracts has been considered sufficient to recover some locomotor function.[24] Repetitive and adequate afferent stimulus, however, is needed to induce a functional gait pattern.[25] To achieve this therapeutic goal, robotic devices have become increasingly important for their capacity to deliver consistent, subject-specific, prolonged training in a safe environment. In this context, lower limb robotic devices have been successfully used in gait rehabilitation after SCI, but studies have not demonstrated their superiority over traditional therapy; hence, their role as an adjunct therapy modality in clinical settings needs further verifications.[26,27]

Similarly, the use of robotic devices in upper extremity rehabilitation in persons with cervical SCI has gained increasing research interest in an effort to achieve behavioral benefits via facilitation of neuroplasticity mechanisms.[28] To date, however, only a few research centers have studied the effects of upper limb robotic training after SCI. Upper limb robotic devices have been used primarily in stroke rehabilitation.[29,30] Many robotic devices have been proposed primarily for use in motor rehabilitation of arm and hand functions of stroke patients and later introduced for use in other neurologic diseases with sensorimotor impairments, such as multiple sclerosis,[31–33] cerebral palsy,[34,35] and Parkinson disease.[36] There are a variety of upper extremity robotic systems that can be divided into 2 main categories: exoskeletons and end-effector robots. Robots, such as MIT-MANUS,[37] Assisted Rehabilitation and Measurement Guide,[38] and Bi-Manu-Track[39] therapy robots, are examples of end-effector robots where patient-robot contact (hand or forearm) is at the end-effector level, and a force is generated at the interface. The MIT-MANUS allows patients to perform reaching movement in the horizontal plane. Exoskeletal robots, on the other hand, are wearable robotic devices that have joint axes that match human anatomic joint axes. Therefore, the joints can be moved in isolation or in synergy in a predetermined movement pattern and torques at each joint can be controlled separately. This allows therapists more flexibility in designing patient-specific treatment protocols. ARMin III,[40] Armeo-Power (the commercial version of the ARMin III),[41] IntelliArm,[42] and EXO-UL7[43] are examples of exoskeleton-based robotic therapy devices. Recently, robot-assisted movement training has been recommended by the American Heart Association/American Stroke Association guidelines for stroke rehabilitation.[44]

As reported in previous studies, robot-aided training is emerging as an adjunct modality for various reasons. First, it can deliver labor-intensive, task-specific exercises at high intensities, for extended periods of time, in a consistent and precise manner. Second, real-time quantified measurement of performance may provide advantages to therapists to modify the therapy protocol based on improvement in performance and monitor motor functions. Third, therapy programs can be automated or semiautomated and not require a close supervision or support from physical/occupational therapist. Potentially, these could be delivered as home therapy programs as devices become smaller, more portable, and less expensive. Fourth, therapy efficiency can be increased with the possibility of group therapy.

ASSESSMENT OF LITERATURE: ROBOTIC-ASSISTED TREATMENT PROTOCOLS

A systematic literature search was conducted in PubMed and Embase using the MeSH terms, "spinal cord injury, upper extremity, rehabilitation, robotics, exoskeleton, end effector." Articles with human subject studies and full text were included without restriction, with publication dates prior to June 26, 2018. This primary search was conducted by a senior librarian and yielded 397 citations. Because the number of literature reports are limited, the authors used an approach similar to that of Singh and colleagues[28] and included all full-text randomized controlled trials (RCTs), case studies, case series, and pre–post design studies in this review. In all studies, robotic device was used as an intervention to improve arm and hand functions.

For initial selection, the abstracts were screened and identified as relevant, irrelevant, or possibly relevant. Then the studies were excluded that were ranked as irrelevant and did not meet inclusion criteria; 15 articles were identified as relevant and the following information extracted:

1. Participant demographics, sample size, dropout rate, time since injury, level of injury, and severity of injury
2. Aim of and information about therapy dosage, type of robot device, duration of study, number of sessions, duration of each session, outcome measure, and conclusion

The objectives and participants' main characteristics of the studies included in this review are presented in **Table 1**.

The type of therapy, targeted body parts, training dosage, and study outcomes are shown in **Table 2**.

Study Participants

A total of 88 participants were enrolled; 80% of the studies enrolled chronic patients and 20% enrolled subacute patients. The average time since injury varied across the studies and ranged between 26 days and 20 years. Injury level ranged from C2 to C7 and included both motor complete (American Spinal Injury Association Impairment Scale [AIS] A–B) and incomplete injuries (AIS C–D); 87% of participants completed the studies whereas the highest dropout rate (2 of 5 participants) in studies at an outpatient setting was related to health issues unrelated to the training.[53] On the other hand, busy schedules, lack of interest, and secondary health complications were cited as reasons for dropout in an inpatient setting.[47] Logistical reasons,[57] long commute time, and secondary medical problems as well as lack of caregiver[58] were named among other reasons. Nevertheless, none of the reasons was related to the intervention per se. Given the rule of thumb that up to 20% of dropouts during a clinical trial can be considered acceptable,[60] a majority of studies did not exceed this rate.

In studies other than case reports, main inclusion criteria were traumatic SCI at cervical level, presence of impaired motor function, tolerance to sitting upright for at least

Table 1
Objectives and characteristics of participants

Study, Year (Ref)	Study Design	Aim	n (n Drop out)	Gender, Age	Spinal Cord Injury Stage	Time Since Injury	Level of Injury
Yozbatiran et al,[45] 2011	Case study	To demonstrate feasibility and effectiveness of robotic training of forearm and wrist movement	1	M, 24 y	Chronic	6.5 mo	C4, AIS D
Kadivar et al,[46] 2011	Case study	To demonstrate safety and effectiveness of robotic training to gain better control of arm and hands	1	M, 24 y	Chronic	6.5 mo	C4, AIS D
Zariffa et al,[47] 2012	Case series	To investigate the use of an upper limb robotic rehabilitation device in subacute cervical SCI	15 (3)	14 M and 1 F, 19–75 y	Subacute	21–173 d	C4–C6, AIS A (2), B (4), C (1), D (5)
Siedziewski et al,[48] 2012	Case study	To study effects of combined robotic and occupational therapy to treat upper extremity dysfunction in tetraplegic patients	1	51 y	Subacute	26 d	C4, AIS D
Yozbatiran et al,[49] 2012	Case study	To evaluate effectiveness of a robotic-assisted training protocol in incomplete tetraplegia	1	F, 28 y	Chronic	29 mo	C2, AIS C
Kadivar et al,[50] 2012	Case series	To test the feasibility of a newly developed robotic device in adults with tetraplegia	2	M and F, 24 y and 27 y	Chronic	6.5, 29 mo	C2, C4 AIS C and D
Cortes et al,[51] 2013	Case series	To evaluate the feasibility, safety and effectiveness of robotic-assisted training in chronic SCI	10	8 M and 2 F, 17–70 y	Chronic	2–8 y	C4–C6 AIS A (3), B (4), C (1), D (2)
Pehlivan et al,[52] 2014	Case study	To validate clinical feasibility and effectiveness of a robotic exoskeleton designed to train forearm and wrist movements	1	M, 45 y	Chronic	83 mo	C3–C5, AIS C

(continued on next page)

Table 1
(continued)

Study, Year (Ref)	Study Design	Aim	n (n Drop out)	Gender, Age	Spinal Cord Injury Stage	Time Since Injury	Level of Injury
Vanmulken et al,[53] 2015	Case series	To test the feasibility of haptic robot technology, and evaluate participants motivation and expectations to work with robot technology	5 (2)	3 M, 25–45 y	Chronic	3.5–11.5 y	C3–C7 AIS A (1), B (2)
Fitle et al,[54] 2015	Case series	To validate clinical feasibility and effectiveness of a robotic exoskeleton designed to train elbow, forearm and wrist movements.	10 (2)	8 M and 2 F, NR	Chronic	NR	C2–C6, AIS C–D
Yozbatiran et al,[55] 2016	RCT	To investigate effectiveness and safety of combined cortical and peripheral stimulation via anodal transcranial direct current stimulation and robotic-assisted training	9 (1)	7M, 1F, 36–62 y	Chronic	7–244 mo	C3–C7, AIS C (3), D (5)
Hoei et al,[56] 2017	Case study	To investigate effects of combined reaching robot with CNMES and FVS to improve shoulder and elbow movements.	1	M, 66 y	Subacute	3 mo	C3–C6 AIS NR
Frullo et al,[57] 2017	Parallel group controlled trial	To study feasibility of subject-adaptive therapy, that is, AAN vs ST modality	17 (3)	12 M and 2 F, mean 53.5 y	Chronic	Mean 16 y	C3–C8, AIS C–D
Francisco et al,[58] 2017	Case series	To demonstrate feasibility, tolerability and effectiveness of robotic-assisted arm training	10 (2)	8 M and 2 F, 19–76 y	Chronic	Mean 49 mo	C2–C7 AIS C (4), D (4)
Yozbatiran et al,[59] 2017	Case series	To investigate relationship between motor recovery and changes in white matter integrity in response to combination therapy	4	3 M and 1 F, 36–63 y	Chronic	8–202 mo	AIS C (1), D (3)

Abbreviations: F, female; M, male; NR, not reported.

Table 2
Type of therapy, targeted arm parts, dosage, and outcomes

Study, Year (Ref.)	Type of Robotic Device	Trained Body Part	Duration	Frequency of Sessions	Duration of Therapy/Session	Robotic Training Stand-alone or in Combination	Outcome Measure	Conclusion
Yozbatiran et al,[45] 2011	Exoskeleton (RiceWrist)	Forearm: pronation/supination, Wrist: flexion/extension, radial/ulnar deviation	2 wk	5 d/wk	180 min (right and left extremities)	Stand-alone	UEMS, grip and pinch strength, JTHFT, FIM	Improvements in pinch strength and hand function. Increased tenodesis effect may play a role.
Kadivar et al,[46] 2011	Exoskeleton RiceWrist	Forearm: pronation/supination, Wrist: flexion/extension, radial/ulnar deviation	2 wk	5 d/wk	180 min (right and left extremities)	Stand-alone	Movement smoothness factor, JTHFT	Less impaired arm demonstrated bigger improvement in movement smoothness and hand function.
Zariffa et al,[47] 2012	Exoskeleton Armeo Spring	Shoulder flexion/extension, abduction/adduction, internal/external rotation; elbow flexion/extension; forearm pronation/supination	6 wk	3–5 days/wk	60 min	Combined with standard occupational and physical therapy exercises	GRASSP, ARAT, grip strength, ROM	GRASSP sensibility showed improvement after treatment and did not maintained at 6 wk

(continued on next page)

Table 2
(continued)

Study, Year (Ref.)	Type of Robotic Device	Trained Body Part	Duration	Frequency of Sessions	Duration of Therapy/Session	Robotic Training Stand-alone or in Combination	Outcome Measure	Conclusion
Siedziewski et al,[48] 2012	End-effector Reo Go[50]	Forward reaching: shoulder abduction/ flexion; forward thrust: shoulder flexion, elbow flexion/ extension; horizontal reach: shoulder abduction, flexion and elbow flexion/ extension; hand to mouth: shoulder flexion, elbow flexion/ extension	20 consecutive days except weekends	5 d/wk	60 min	Stand-alone	AROM, FIM, CUE	Increase in AROM and strength, increase in independence in self-care, increase in perceived UE function
Yozbatiran et al,[49] 2012	Exoskeleton MAHI Exo-II	Elbow flexion/ extension, forearm pronation/ supination, wrist flexion/extension and radial/ulnar deviation	4 wk	3 d/wk	180 min (right and left extremities)	Stand-alone	UEMS, ARAT, JTHFT, safety measures	Bigger improvement in hand functions on the less impaired side. No excessive fatigue, pain, and discomfort.
Kadivar et al,[50] 2012	Exoskeleton RiceWrist	forearm pronation/ supination, wrist flexion/ extension and radial/ulnar deviation	Case 1: 7 sessions, case 2: 10 sessions	Case 1: N/A case 2: 5 d/wk	60–180 min (right and left extremities)	Stand-alone	Movement smoothness, JTHFT	Noticeable improvements in movement smoothness on the stronger arm and hand functions

Study	Device	Movement/Training	Duration	Frequency	Time	Mode	Outcome Measures	Results
Cortes et al,[51] 2013	Exoskeleton InMotion 3.0 Wrist robot	Forearm pronation/supination, Wrist flexion/extension	6 wk	3 times[51]	1 h/d	Stand-alone	Robot-measured kinematics, corticospinal excitability, motor strength, pain and spasticity	No adverse effects. Significant improvements in motor performance kinematics, and movement smoothness. No change in muscle strength and corticospinal excitability.
Pehlivan et al,[52] 2014	Exoskeleton RiceWrist-S	Forearm pronation/supination, wrist flexion/extension	20 d	10 sessions[53]	53	Stand-alone	UEMS, JTHFT, ARAT pinch and grip force Movement smoothness	Improvement in JTHFT, ARAT, grip force. No changes in muscle strength.
Vanmulken et al,[53] 2015	End-effector Haptic Master	Goal dependent functional and client-specific skill training	6 wk	3 d/wk	60 min	Combined with task-oriented training	USE, IMI, CEQ, AHF, SCIM, muscle strength, function level	Working with the robotic device was easy to learn and perform. No significant improvement in SCIM, activity level. Sparse improvement for muscle strength.

(continued on next page)

Table 2
(continued)

Study, Year (Ref.)	Type of Robotic Device	Trained Body Part	Duration	Frequency of Sessions	Duration of Therapy/Session	Robotic Training Stand-alone or in Combination	Outcome Measure	Conclusion
Fitle et al,[54] 2015	Exoskeleton MAHI Exo-II	Elbow flexion/extension, forearm pronation/supination, wrist flexion/extension and radial/ulnar deviation	4 wk	2–3 d/wk	180 min (right and left extremities)	Stand-alone	Robotic data assessment measures, JTHFT, ARAT	Robotic measure improved significantly in the less affected limb.
Yozbatiran et al,[55] 2016	Exoskeleton MAHI Exo-II	Elbow flexion/extension, forearm pronation/supination, wrist flexion/extension and radial/ulnar deviation	2 wk	5 d/wk	60 min	Combined with cortical stimulation	UEMS, JTHFT, MAS, MAL-AOU	All participants in the active and sham stimulation groups tended to perform better in JTHFT, AOU-MAL. Improvement in hand functions was higher in active stimulation group.
Hoei et al,[56] 2017	End-effector Reaching Robot	Upper limb reaching[57]	8 wk with 4 wk of robotic training	7 d/wk	20 min	Combined with distal RFE	SIAS, STEF, AROM, MAS	Upper extremity function improved on all outcome measures except for MAS of the wrist extensor

Study	Device	Joints/Motions	Duration	Frequency	Session	Mode	Outcome measures	Results
Frullo et al,[57] 2017	Exoskeleton MAHI Exo-II	Elbow flexion/extension, forearm pronation/supination, wrist flexion/extension and radial/ulnar deviation	4 wk	1–3 d/wk (total 10 sessions)	90 min	Stand-alone	Robotic data movement quality, ARAT, GRASSP	AAN provided greater increase in movement quality over the ST controller. No significant change in ARAT score.
Francisco et al,[58] 2017	Exoskeleton MAHI Exo-II	Elbow flexion/extension, forearm pronation/supination, wrist flexion/extension and radial/ulnar deviation	4 wk	3 d/wk	180 min (right and left extremities)	Stand-alone	UEMS, JTHFT, ARAT, grip and pinch strength, SCIM	Improved arm and hand functions. Independence in daily life has not changed. No adverse events.
Yozbatiran et al,[59] 2017	Exoskeleton MAHI Exo-II	Elbow flexion/extension, forearm pronation/supination, wrist flexion/extension and radial/ulnar deviation	2 wk	5 d/wk	60 min	Combined with cortical stimulation	DTI metrics, JTHFT, MAL-AOU	DTI metrics shown positive change in both groups. Greater improvement in active group compared with sham stimulation group.

Abbreviations: AOU-MAL, amount of use-motor activity log; AROM, active range of motion; CEQ, credibility and expectancy questionnaire; CUE, capabilities of upper extremity instrument; DTI, diffusion tensor imaging; FIM, functional independence measure; GRASSP, graded and redefined assessment of strength, sensibility, and prehension; IMI, intrinsic motivation inventory; JTHFT, Jebsen-Taylor hand function test; MAHI, mechatronics and haptic interfaces lab; MAS, modified ashworth scale; SCIM, spinal cord independence measure; SIAS, stroke impairment assessment set; STEF, simple test for evaluating hand function; UEMS, upper extremity motor score; USE, usefulness, satisfaction and ease-of-use questionnaire.

1 hour, no previous central or peripheral nervous system insult interfering with interpretation of the results, cognitive ability sufficient to cooperate with the intervention, and no joint contracture of severe spasticity in the affected upper limb as measured by a Modified Ashworth Scale score of higher than 3 out of 4. Exclusion criteria were presence of progressive neurodegenerative disorder, concomitant traumatic brain injury or stroke, uncontrolled pain in the affected limb or exercise intolerance, ongoing use of CNS active medications, and not being able to provide self-transportation. In addition, 3 studies excluded participants if they demonstrated contraindication to transcranial magnetic stimulation[51] and transcranial direct current stimulation (tDCS)[55] as well as MRI.[59]

Of the 15 included articles, 6 were case studies, 7 were case series, 1 was a parallel group controlled trial, and 1 was a randomized clinical trial (RCT). None of the studies used usual care as control group; therefore, a true comparison of robotic-assisted training with standard occupational therapy programs cannot be drawn from review. Only 1 study used the opposite arm as a control, in which participants received standard occupational and physical therapy exercises during the course of study.[47]

Type of robotic devices in the included studies were either exoskeleton or end-effector devices. The exoskeleton-type devices were RiceWrist,[45,46,50] Armeo Spring (Hocoma, Switzerland),[47] MAHI Exo-II,[49,54,55,57–59] InMotion 3.0 Wrist Robot (Bionik, USA),[51] and RiceWrist-S,[52] and the end-effector devices used in the studies were ReoGo (Motorika Inc., USA)[48] and Haptic Master (Moog, Nieuw-Vennep, The Netherlands).[53]

The clinical effects of robotic-assisted arm training were evaluated with muscle strength, active range of motion, muscle tonus, arm and hand functions, grip and pinch strength, amount of use in daily tasks, and independence in daily life. A few studies also used robotic measures to capture changes in movement quality: number of peaks, velocity profile of a given movement, normalized mean speed, and smoothness correlation coefficient, which were extracted from data collected during robotic training sessions and analyzed off-line.[46,51,52,54,57]

All study protocols were supervised. Although robotic-assisted training was performed stand-alone in a majority of studies, 2 studies investigated effects of combined treatment protocols. In these studies, robotic-assisted training was combined with stimulation of primary motor cortex via anodal tDCS, a method of noninvasive brain stimulation. Anodal tDCS was used to enhance cortical excitability prior to repetitive training. Participants who received sham stimulation served as a control group.[55] In another study, robotic therapy was combined with peripheral stimulation via continuous low-amplitude neuromuscular electrical stimulation (CNMES) and functional vibratory stimulation.[56]

An overview of the training parameters of each intervention is given in **Table 2**. Overall, treatment dosage (ie, treatment length [duration], frequency of sessions, number of total sessions, and duration of each session) varied between studies. The duration of treatment programs ranged from 2 weeks (wk) to 6 weeks, with a frequency ranging from 1 d/wk to 5 d/wk and a session duration of 20 minutes to 180 minutes. Although the training protocols were performed in a set of repetitions of single joint movements or repetitive task training, only a few studies reported the actual number of repetitions.[48,49] The body parts involved in training were localized to single joint or involved the whole arm, including shoulder movements. The duration of each session included set-up, donning and doffing the device, adjusting settings, and giving intermittent breaks to avoid excessive fatigue that may rise from high-intensity repetitive training. None of the included studies included information about actual training time.

Table 2 gives an overview of body parts involved in the training and treatment dosage.

Effectiveness

The efficacy of robot-assisted training on arm and hand functions, independence in daily life, and movement quality seems positive but with sparse results. Studies reported increased muscle strength,[45,48,49,53,55,58] active range of motion,[48,56] arm and hand function,[45,47–51,53,56,58,59] and pinch and grip strength.[49,52,57,58] Positive changes in movement quality[50–52,57] and corticospinal tract structure[59] were demonstrated in other studies. Corticospinal excitability[51] and sensory function[48] did not show significant change after therapy.

Although safety issues were not systematically reported in the included studies, overall there were no complications or major adverse events during or after robotic-assisted arm training. In addition, all dropouts were unrelated to the treatment protocol. Only 1 subject indicated lack of interest[47] but there is no further information whether the subject declined participation due to lack of interest in training with a robotic device per se or more generally was not interested in participating in a research study.

Discussion

Major advances in rehabilitation technologies have occurred over the past 2 decades, with development and testing of robotic devices in rehabilitation of motor impairments. This literature assessment provides an overview of robotic-assisted training protocols used for improving arm and hand functions after cervical SCI. Despite the low number of included studies, results from the included studies suggest that robotic training protocols are feasible and well tolerated and have a positive impact on improving arm and hand functions in a select group of patients with cervical SCI, but the results must be interpreted with caution. Because testing of robotic-assisted arm training as a treatment modality in this population is still in its infancy, there is substantial need for feasibility assessments that will provide important insight in understanding this new strategy. Before using large amounts of resources to study effectiveness of robotic-assisted training in phase III trials, more phase II studies are needed to provide sound evidence in understanding clinical validity of specific robotic devices, treatment dosages, and characteristics of responders with cervical SCI to robotic-assisted therapy.

From a clinical standpoint, robotic devices should be designed to allow repetitive movement practice at high intensities, be equipped with a controller that provides the least assistance needed to accomplish the movement/task (assist-as-needed [AAN]), provide reproducible treatment protocols, and provide an interactive form of task training. Consistent with evidence that activity produces plastic changes in the CNS and enhances motor learning,[61] recovery relies heavily on a patient's active engagement in therapy. Most of the upper limb robots have the capacity to passively move the extremity through prescribed trajectories, but this form of training is not likely to be efficacious and hence not desired by occupational or physical therapists.

Adaptive robotic training protocols[62] may have the potential to fill this gap in interaction algorithms between patient and robotic device. Ideally, treatment protocols should challenge the patient to actively engage throughout the movement and provide assistance only when needed (AAN). Among included articles, the only study testing effects of 2 different robotic controllers on arm and hand function in cervical SCI was by Frullo and colleagues.[57] In this study, the investigators compared an AAN controller to adjust challenge and robotic assistance continuously during movement with a nonadaptive subject-triggered (ST) controller. With the ST control approach, a therapist adjusted the challenge of treatment delivery, manually controlling the force threshold for initiation the movement via a graphical user interface. After 10 sessions of robotic training of elbow and wrist movements, patients did not demonstrate significant difference in arm and hand functions as measured with the Action Research Arm Test (ARAT). Movement quality improved in both groups, and although the AAN group demonstrated consistent improvement across all joint movements and all robotic measures of movement quality, the ST group showed smaller gains confined to only a subset of the metrics and joint movements.

Well-designed robot-assisted rehabilitation research studies also should incorporate outcome measures that are reliable, repeatable, valid, and sensitive to detect small changes in function.

The International Classification of Functioning, Disability and Health can be a useful guide because diseases and conditions are often categorized into measurement of body functions and structure, activities, and participation.[2] For example, outcome measurements not only should focus on body function/structure (joint range of motion, muscle strength, and muscle tonus) but also include more complex activities with the arm and hand, such as dressing, eating, washing, preparation of meals, and so forth.[63] Thus, engineers and clinicians will have a better understanding of each other's expectations from an intervention that is primarily designed to improve patients' arm and hand functions to optimize their capacity at activity and participation levels. For example, improving muscle strength or active range of motion (body functions and structures) may not necessarily translate into improved activity level; thus, patients may not perform better in eating, dressing, and so forth. This classification also will assist in optimizing treatment protocols.

Recovery after SCI is a long and complex process, and clinical and functional measures may fail to capture small changes related to spontaneous recovery and/or treatment-induced recovery during acute, subacute, or chronic stages. Fortunately, robotic systems have the capability to extract movement kinematics that can provide precise information about movement quality, such as deviation from a given trajectory, average speed, peak speed, and smoothness of movement, that otherwise may not be reflected in functional measurements.

Overall, articles included in this review demonstrated wide variation in the amount of treatment (including duration, frequency, and number of movement repetitions), type of treatment (stand-alone or combinations with other treatments targeting peripheral muscular training or enhancing motor cortex neuronal activity), and study populations. In addition, the clinical applicability of the robotic training needs to be confirmed in well-designed, dose-matched, RCTs with larger sample size and long-term follow-up.

SUMMARY

Dose-matched, randomized, phase II clinical trials are needed to optimize treatment protocols that aim to promote recovery of upper limb movements within the context of facilitating neural networks at spinal and supraspinal level, thereby inducing intrinsic recovery mechanism and improving functions.

Given the strong evidence from both clinical practice and research, individuals with tetraplegia have a great desire to improve control of their arm and hand functions. This evidence should lead rehabilitation researchers to combine their effort with engineers and neuroscientists to design and develop treatment protocols with optimized frequency, intensity, and duration and type of training.

REFERENCES

1. National Spinal Cord Injury Statistical Center. Spinal cord injury facts and figures at a glance. Birmingham (AL): University of Alabama Birmingham; 2018. p. 2.

2. Herrmann KH, Kirchberger I, Biering-Sorensen F, et al. Differences in functioning of individuals with tetraplegia and paraplegia according to the International Classification of Functioning, Disability and Health (ICF). Spinal Cord 2011;49(4): 534–43.

3. Brogioli M, Schneider S, Popp WL, et al. Monitoring upper limb recovery after cervical spinal cord injury: insights beyond assessment scores. Front Neurol 2016;7: 142.

4. Anderson KD. Targeting recovery: priorities of the spinal cord-injured population. J Neurotrauma 2004;21(10):1371–83.

5. Snoek GJ, Ijzerman MJ, Hermens HJ, et al. Survey of the needs of patients with spinal cord injury: impact and priority for improvement in hand function in tetraplegics. Spinal cord 2004;42(9):526–32.

6. Rudhe C, van Hedel HJ. Upper extremity function in persons with tetraplegia: relationships between strength, capacity, and the spinal cord independence measure. Neurorehabil Neural Repair 2009;23(5):413–21.

7. Ramón y Cajal S, May RM. Degeneration & regeneration of the nervous system. London: Oxford University Press, Humphrey Milford; 1928.

8. Bunday KL, Perez MA. Motor recovery after spinal cord injury enhanced by strengthening corticospinal synaptic transmission. Curr Biol 2012;22(24): 2355–61.

9. Ding Y, Kastin AJ, Pan W. Neural plasticity after spinal cord injury. Curr Pharm Des 2005;11(11):1441–50.

10. Popovic MR, Kapadia N, Zivanovic V, et al. Functional electrical stimulation therapy of voluntary grasping versus only conventional rehabilitation for patients with subacute incomplete tetraplegia: a randomized clinical trial. Neurorehabil Neural Repair 2011;25(5):433–42.

11. Walker HW, Lee MY, Bahroo LB, et al. Botulinum toxin injection techniques for the management of adult spasticity. PM R 2015;7(4):417–27.

12. Kilgore KL, Hoyen HA, Bryden AM, et al. An implanted upper-extremity neuroprosthesis using myoelectric control. J Hand Surg Am 2008;33(4):539–50.

13. Ortner R, Allison BZ, Korisek G, et al. An SSVEP BCI to control a hand orthosis for persons with tetraplegia. IEEE Trans Neural Syst Rehabil Eng 2011;19(1):1–5.

14. Hamou C, Shah NR, DiPonio L, et al. Pinch and elbow extension restoration in people with tetraplegia: a systematic review of the literature. J Hand Surg Am 2009;34(4):692–9.

15. Kleim JA, Jones TA. Principles of experience-dependent neural plasticity: implications for rehabilitation after brain damage. J Speech Lang Hear Res 2008; 51(1):S225–39.

16. Krebs HI, Volpe BT. Rehabilitation robotics. Handb Clin Neurol 2013;110:283–94.

17. Lo K, Stephenson M, Lockwood C. Effectiveness of robotic assisted rehabilitation for mobility and functional ability in adult stroke patients: a systematic review. JBI Database Syst Rev Implement Rep 2017;15(12):3049–91.

18. Reinkensmeyer DJ, Boninger ML. Technologies and combination therapies for enhancing movement training for people with a disability. J Neuroeng Rehabil 2012;9:17.

19. Reinkensmeyer DJ, Wolbrecht ET, Chan V, et al. Comparison of three-dimensional, assist-as-needed robotic arm/hand movement training provided with Pneu-WREX to conventional tabletop therapy after chronic stroke. Am J Phys Med Rehabil 2012;91(11 Suppl 3):S232–41.

20. Kutner NG, Zhang R, Butler AJ, et al. Quality-of-life change associated with robotic-assisted therapy to improve hand motor function in patients with sub-acute stroke: a randomized clinical trial. Phys Ther 2010;90(4):493–504.

21. Takahashi CD, Der-Yeghiaian L, Le V, et al. Robot-based hand motor therapy after stroke. Brain 2008;131(Pt 2):425–37.

22. Volpe BT, Lynch D, Rykman-Berland A, et al. Intensive sensorimotor arm training mediated by therapist or robot improves hemiparesis in patients with chronic stroke. Neurorehabil Neural Repair 2008;22(3):305–10.

23. de Leon RD, Hodgson JA, Roy RR, et al. Locomotor capacity attributable to step training versus spontaneous recovery after spinalization in adult cats. J Neurophysiol 1998;79(3):1329–40.

24. Basso DM. Neuroanatomical substrates of functional recovery after experimental spinal cord injury: implications of basic science research for human spinal cord injury. Phys Ther 2000;80(8):808–17.

25. Dietz V. Body weight supported gait training: from laboratory to clinical setting. Brain Res Bull 2008;76(5):459–63.

26. Holanda LJ, Silva PMM, Amorim TC, et al. Robotic assisted gait as a tool for reha-bilitation of individuals with spinal cord injury: a systematic review. J Neuroeng Rehabil 2017;14(1):126.

27. Mehrholz J, Harvey LA, Thomas S, et al. Is body-weight-supported treadmill training or robotic-assisted gait training superior to overground gait training and other forms of physiotherapy in people with spinal cord injury? A systematic review. Spinal Cord 2017;55(8):722–9.

28. Singh H, Unger J, Zariffa J, et al. Robot-assisted upper extremity rehabilitation for cervical spinal cord injuries: a systematic scoping review. Disabil Rehabil Assist Technol 2018;13(7):704–15.

29. Lo AC, Guarino PD, Richards LG, et al. Robot-assisted therapy for long-term up-per-limb impairment after stroke. N Engl J Med 2010;362(19):1772–83.

30. Mehrholz J, Hadrich A, Platz T, et al. Electromechanical and robot-assisted arm training for improving generic activities of daily living, arm function, and arm mus-cle strength after stroke. Cochrane Database Syst Rev 2012;(6):CD006876.

31. Carpinella I, Cattaneo D, Abuarqub S, et al. Robot-based rehabilitation of the up-per limbs in multiple sclerosis: feasibility and preliminary results. J Rehabil Med 2009;41(12):966–70.

32. Feys P, Coninx K, Kerkhofs L, et al. Robot-supported upper limb training in a vir-tual learning environment : a pilot randomized controlled trial in persons with MS. J Neuroeng Rehabil 2015;12:60.

33. Gijbels D, Lamers I, Kerkhofs L, et al. The Armeo Spring as training tool to improve upper limb functionality in multiple sclerosis: a pilot study. J Neuroeng Rehabil 2011;8:5.

34. Fasoli SE, Fragala-Pinkham M, Hughes R, et al. Upper limb robotic therapy for children with hemiplegia. Am J Phys Med Rehabil 2008;87(11):929–36.

35. Picelli A, La Marchina E, Vangelista A, et al. Effects of robot-assisted training for the unaffected arm in patients with hemiparetic cerebral palsy: a proof-of-concept pilot study. Behav Neurol 2017;2017:8349242.

36. Picelli A, Tamburin S, Passuello M, et al. Robot-assisted arm training in patients with Parkinson's disease: a pilot study. J Neuroeng Rehabil 2014;11:28.

37. Krebs HI, Volpe BT, Williams D, et al. Robot-aided neurorehabilitation: a robot for wrist rehabilitation. IEEE Trans Neural Syst Rehabil Eng 2007;15(3):327–35.

38. Reinkensmeyer DJ, Kahn LE, Averbuch M, et al. Understanding and treating arm movement impairment after chronic brain injury: progress with the ARM guide. J Rehabil Res Dev 2000;37(6):653–62.
39. Hesse S, Werner C, Pohl M, et al. Computerized arm training improves the motor control of the severely affected arm after stroke: a single-blinded randomized trial in two centers. Stroke 2005;36(9):1960–6.
40. Nef T, Guidali M, Riener R. ARMin III- arm therapy exoskeleton with an ergonomic shoulder actuation. Appl Bionics Biomech 2009;6(2):127–42.
41. Riener R, Guidali M, Keller U, et al. Transferring armin to the clinics and industry. Top Spinal Cord Inj Rehabil 2011;17:54–9.
42. Ren Y, Kang SH, Park HS, et al. Developing a multi-joint upper limb exoskeleton robot for diagnosis, therapy, and outcome evaluation in neurorehabilitation. IEEE Trans Neural Syst Rehabil Eng 2013;21(3):490–9.
43. Simkins M, Kim H, Abrams G, et al. Robotic unilateral and bilateral upper-limb movement training for stroke survivors afflicted by chronic hemiparesis. IEEE Int Conf Rehabil Robot 2013;2013:6650506.
44. Winstein CJ, Stein J, Arena R, et al, American Heart Association Stroke Council, Council on Cardiovascular and Stroke Nursing, Council on Clinical Cardiology, Council on Quality of Care and Outcomes Research. Guidelines for adult stroke rehabilitation and recovery: a guideline for healthcare professionals from the American Heart Association/American Stroke Association. Stroke 2016;47(6): e98–169.
45. Yozbatiran N, Berliner J, Boake C, et al. Robotic training and clinical assessment of forearm and wrist movements after incomplete spinal cord injury: a case study. IEEE Int Conf Rehabil Robot 2011;2011:5975425.
46. Kadivar Z, Sullivan JL, Eng DP, et al. Robotic training and kinematic analysis of arm and hand after incomplete spinal cord injury: a case study. IEEE Int Conf Rehabil Robot 2011;2011:5975429.
47. Zariffa J, Kapadia N, Kramer JL, et al. Feasibility and efficacy of upper limb robotic rehabilitation in a subacute cervical spinal cord injury population. Spinal Cord 2012;50(3):220–6.
48. Siedziewski L, Schaaf RC, Mount J. Use of robotics in spinal cord injury: a case report. Am J Occup Ther 2012;66(1):51–8.
49. Yozbatiran N, Berliner J, O'Malley MK, et al. Robotic training and clinical assessment of upper extremity movements after spinal cord injury: a single case report. J Rehabil Med 2012;44(2):186–8.
50. Kadivar Z, Sullivan JL, Pehlivan AU, et al. RiceWrist robotic device for upper limb training: feasibility study and case report of two tetraplegic persons with spinal cord. Int J Biol Eng 2012;2(4):27–38.
51. Cortes M, Elder J, Rykman A, et al. Improved motor performance in chronic spinal cord injury following upper-limb robotic training. NeuroRehabilitation 2013; 33(1):57–65.
52. Pehlivan AU, Sergi F, Erwin A, et al. Design and validation of the RiceWrist-S exoskeleton for robotic rehabilitation after incomplete spinal cord injury. Robotica 2014;32:1415–31.
53. Vanmulken DA, Spooren AI, Bongers HM, et al. Robot-assisted task-oriented upper extremity skill training in cervical spinal cord injury: a feasibility study. Spinal Cord 2015;53(7):547–51.
54. Fitle KD, Pehlivan AU, O'Malley MK. A Robotic Exoskeleton for rehabilitation and assessment of the upper limb following incomplete spinal cord injury IEEE

International Conference on Robotics and Automation, Seattle, May 26-30, 2015, p. 4960–6.

55. Yozbatiran N, Keser Z, Davis M, et al. Transcranial direct current stimulation (tDCS) of the primary motor cortex and robot-assisted arm training in chronic incomplete cervical spinal cord injury: a proof of concept sham-randomized clinical study. NeuroRehabilitation 2016;39(3):401–11.

56. Hoei T, Kawahira K, Fukuda H, et al. Use of an arm weight-bearing combined with upper-limb reaching apparatus to facilitate motor paralysis recovery in an incomplete spinal cord injury patient: a single case report. J Phys Ther Sci 2017;29(1): 176–80.

57. Frullo JM, Elinger J, Pehlivan AU, et al. Effects of assist-as-needed upper extremity robotic therapy after incomplete spinal cord injury: a parallel-group controlled trial. Front Neurorobot 2017;11:26.

58. Francisco GE, Yozbatiran N, Berliner J, et al. Robot-assisted training of arm and hand movement shows functional improvements for incomplete cervical spinal cord injury. Am J Phys Med Rehabil 2017;96(10 Suppl 1):S171–7.

59. Yozbatiran N, Keser Z, Hasan K, et al. White matter changes in corticospinal tract associated with improvement in arm and hand functions in incomplete cervical spinal cord injury: pilot case series. Spinal Cord Ser Cases 2017;3:17028.

60. Furlan AD, Pennick V, Bombardier C, et al. 2009 updated method guidelines for systematic reviews in the Cochrane Back Review Group. Spine (Phila Pa 1976) 2009;34(18):1929–41.

61. Warraich Z, Kleim JA. Neural plasticity: the biological substrate for neurorehabilitation. PM R 2010;2(12 Suppl 2):S208–19.

62. Pehlivan AU, Sergi F, O'Malley MK. Adaptive control of a serial-in-parallel robotic rehabilitation device. IEEE Int Conf Rehabil Robot 2013;2013:6650412.

63. World Health Organization. International classification of functioning, disability and health (ICF). World Health Organization: Geneva (Switzerland); 2001.

Robotics for Lower Limb Rehabilitation

Alberto Esquenazi, MD*, Mukul Talaty, PhD

KEYWORDS

- Tethered exoskeletons • End-effector devices • Untethered exoskeletons
- Gait rehabilitation

KEY POINTS

- The pace of development in robotic technologies for gait training continues to increase, as well as become more specialized.
- There generally has been a deepened focus on understanding the active ingredients in robotic therapy, along with a concerted effort to clarify relationships between dose and outcomes.
- More work is needed to define the therapeutic applications of these devices and further technical improvements are expected regarding device size; controls; and, for untethered devices, battery life and portability.

INTRODUCTION

Improving walking function is an important goal of rehabilitation and a primary concern with respect to social and vocational reintegration for a person with neurologic-related gait impairment. Robots for lower limb gait rehabilitation have been designed principally to automate repetitive labor-intensive training and to assist therapists[1] and patients during various stages of neurorehabilitation. Part of this latter mandate includes providing the most beneficial type of activities, not just in number of repetitions, safety, and motivation under which they are performed but also in terms of activities that strike the ideal balance between accuracy and variability of movement, appropriate and precisely adjustable levels of resistance, and optimal unweighting and assistance in performing the movements. The optimal values for these parameters are not known at this time; however, the training paradigms have their roots in theories of motor learning.

Motor learning reflects a neural specificity of practice because motor skill acquisition involves the integration of the sensory and motor information that occurs during practice and, ultimately, leads to a pattern that results in accurate, consistent, and skillful movements. Rehabilitation based on the concepts of repetitive, intensive,

The authors have nothing to disclose.
MossRehab Gait and Motion Analysis Laboratory, 60 Township Line, Elkins Park, PA 19027, USA
* Corresponding author.
E-mail address: AESQUENA@einstein.edu

Phys Med Rehabil Clin N Am 30 (2019) 385–397
https://doi.org/10.1016/j.pmr.2018.12.012
1047-9651/19/© 2018 Elsevier Inc. All rights reserved.

task-oriented training has been shown to be effective. The therapeutic goals of this approach are to achieve restoration and recovery of walking by harnessing the inherent capacities of the spinal and supraspinal locomotor centers.[2] Treadmill training with partial bodyweight support involves supporting some of the patient's weight over a motorized treadmill while clinicians use manual facilitation assistance techniques to produce stepping motions. The technique aims to restore a normal physiologic gait pattern, with attention to the ideal kinematic and temporal aspects of gait.[3] Robotic devices have been designed to reduce the demands of the manual-assistance repetitive task and improve gait performance. Scientific and clinical evidence for the effectiveness, safety, and tolerability of gait training with robotic devices exists; however, documentation of their advantages compared with conventional therapies is limited. This might be due in part to the lack of appropriate patient selection and the parameters of locomotor training interventions choice based on functional impairments. The design of the robot cannot be ruled out as a possible cause. Despite this shortcoming, robotic devices are being integrated into clinical settings with positive results in several applications. Appropriate use depends on the clinician's knowledge of different robotic devices, as well as the ability to use the devices' technical features, thereby allowing patients to benefit from robot-aided gait training throughout the rehabilitation continuum with the ultimate goal of returning to safe and efficient overground walking.

There is increasing evidence to support the concept of reorganization and plasticity of the injured central nervous system (CNS). The potential for reorganization is particularly high early after CNS injury but also possible at later stages.[4–7] Reorganization in a functionally meaningful way seems to depend on motor activity as executed during rehabilitative training and followed by functional improvements.[8,9] The science behind exercise in CNS disorders is supported by the therapy concept of increased dosage effect.[10] Task-oriented, high-repetition movements based on the principles of motor learning can improve, among other things, muscular strength, motor control, and movement coordination in patients with neurologic impairments.[11,12] Gait training can help prevent secondary complications, such as muscle atrophy, osteoporosis, joint stiffness, and muscle and soft tissue shortening, and promotes the reduction of spasticity, among other benefits.[13]

Robots enhance the rehabilitation process and may improve therapeutic outcomes, and have the potential to support clinical evaluation by allowing instrumented measurement of physiologic and performance parameters, precisely control and measure the therapeutic intervention, implement novel forms of mechanical manipulation impossible for therapists to provide, and supply different forms of feedback, thereby increasing patient's motivation and improving outcomes.[2,3,14] Robots for rehabilitation were designed as a clinical tool to automate the labor-intensive repetitive training techniques, especially in the early stage of neurologic recovery in which patients may require a high amount of support. Their programmable force-producing ability allows robotic devices to promote task-oriented movements and provide more correct afferent feedback by guiding the limb to promote heel strike and hip extension during initial contact and midstance of walking. Weight-supported treadmill training unweighs the patient and permits the use of a motorized treadmill for walking. Depending on the patient's abilities and functional capacity, up to 4 therapists may be required to secure and stabilize a patient and guide the trunk and legs through a normal gait trajectory.[15] Robotic technology can increase the duration and number of training sessions while reducing the number of assisting therapists required. Robotic-assisted gait training takes advantage of similar features of unweighing the lower limbs and a motorized treadmill, and substitutes for the manual labor of the therapists with an exoskeleton robotic system that can consistently and reliably position and move the limbs during walking[15] while providing a comparable amount of degrees of freedom for the ankle; knee; and, with recent technical advances, the hip; and range of motion to promote a natural and comfortable gait.[1]

The robotic devices described herein offer training conditions supportive of the principles for the enhancement of neuroplastic changes in patients with CNS-related gait impairment. The principles of intensity, repetition, task specificity, and engagement are met in varying capacities by these training devices. Within the last 15 years, the number of robotic therapy devices for upper and lower extremity rehabilitation has rapidly expanded. For gait training, 4 major robotic categories have been defined:

- Tethered exoskeletons
- End-effector devices
- Untethered exoskeletons
- Patient-guided suspension systems.

Tethered exoskeletal systems, such as the Lokomat (**Fig. 1**) (Hocoma AG, Switzerland),[16] LOPES (University of Twente, Netherlands),[17] and ReoAmbulator (Motorika, New Jersey, USA),[18] apply forces through a rigid articulated frame that move the patient's legs in 1 or more planes in conjunction with a bodyweight support system. End-effector–based systems, such as the Gait Trainer GT II (Reha-Stim, Germany)[19] and G-EO systems (**Fig. 2**) (Reha Technologies, Switzerland),[20] work based on a constraint (ie, force applied) at the distal end of the kinetic chain that specifies the trajectory there and the proximal joints can simply move as the body geometry and articulations dictate. Often, this means the feet are strapped to 2 moving footplates, as in an elliptical trainer, and moved by the device in a gait-like trajectory with less robotic control over the proximal joints.

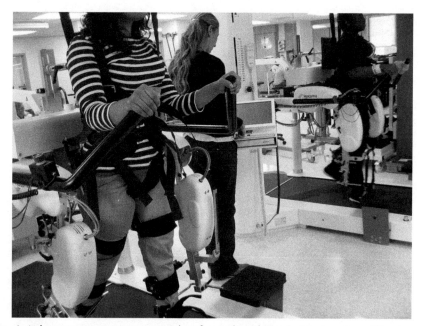

Fig. 1. Lokomat system as an example of a tethered exoskeleton system. (*Courtesy of* MossRehab with permission from Hocoma AG, Switzerland.)

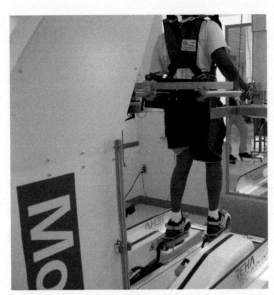

Fig. 2. G-EO Evolution system as an example of an end-effector system. (*Courtesy of* MossRehab with permission from Reha Technologies, Switzerland.)

Untethered exoskeletons, such as the ReWalk (ReWalk Robotics, Inc, Massachusetts, USA), Indego (Parker Hannefin Corp, Ohio, USA), and the Ekso (Ekso Bionics, California, USA) are wearable, powered, articulated suits with self-contained power sources and control algorithms that allow the most freedom and realistic walking experience.

Patient-guided suspension systems are nonanchored robotic walking frames that allow overground, supported walking through a rolling frame with sensors and control algorithms to assist with propulsion and steering of the frame, and provide a harness and/or trunk or pelvic support during walking. An example of these devices is the Andago, Hocoma AG, Switzerland. Although of great potential benefit and less cost, this article will focus primarily on the first 3 categories of devices for which more scientific data and clinical experience are available.[21]

Tethered Exoskeletons

Tethered exoskeletons have a device that surrounds the patient's legs, which may be suspended from an overhead guide rail, supported by a metal frame on wheels, or the exoskeleton can even be directly supported by a mobile robot. Stationary exoskeletons are usually connected directly to the ground through a rigid frame or bolted to a wall, enhancing and ensuring total safety. Stationary and tethered exoskeletons can have large and powerful motors and controllers, with none of their weight transferred to the user. These devices often involve walking on a treadmill. Tethered exoskeletons tend to be somewhat less complex in their engineering design and more stable and inherently safer than devices that permit overground walking owing to the elimination of fall risk. Some devices have control systems that can sense and dynamically adjust performance assistance. One potential limitation of these systems is that they are less accommodating of individual gait variations. Examples of tethered exoskeletons include the Lokomat,[22] WalkTrainer,[23] NaTUre-gaits,[24] LOPES,[17] ReoAmbulator, and the Anklebot.

Some evidence points to the robotic component showing equivalent if not increased effectiveness compared with more conventional physical therapy, while other evidence does not; for example, in the stroke population,[25,26] and confirms the long-standing notion that these devices do lessen the physical demands on the therapists by providing partial bodyweight-supported treadmill training. The largest body of scientific evidence is for the Lokomat when used by individuals with a spinal cord injury (SCI) or stroke. This device is commercially available with a significant installed user base, allowing completion of clinical trials. Despite this, or perhaps because of this, there is no consensus of whether and how it affects outcomes in comparison with conventional or other types of robotic therapy.[1,27-39] Recently published data from the Advanced Robotic Therapy Integrated Centers (ARTIC) network using a pragmatic observational study of clinical care exploit variations in practice to learn about current clinical application of the Lokomat and its outcomes. The database includes patients with various neurologic diagnosis with gait deficits who used the Lokomat as part of their rehabilitation. At time of analysis, the database contained data collected from 595 patients (cerebral palsy, n = 208; stroke, n = 129; SCI, n = 93; traumatic brain injury, n = 39; and various other diagnoses, n = 126). At onset, average walking speeds were slow. The training intensity increased from the first to the final therapy session and most patients achieved their set goals.[40] Other devices, such as the ReoAmbulator, have very limited published reports with similarly conflicting results.[18,41-43] An initial report on LOPES showed improved walking ability, as well as gait quality, in subjects with incomplete SCI after an 8-week treatment program, with slower walking subjects showing greater benefits.[44]

Motivation through a therapeutic gaming interface, possible in all of the systems, increases patient engagement and tolerance to therapy, and reduces perceived discomfort, as demonstrated in pediatric patients with cerebral palsy.[45] Labruyere and colleagues[46] quantified game participation, using electromyographic muscle activity (*Musculus rectus femoris*) and heart rate during a demanding part and a less demanding part of the game. They conclude that children with neurologic gait disorders are able to modify their activity to the demands built into a virtual reality scenario. Cognitive function and motor impairment determine to what extent they can do so.

End-Effector Devices

End-effector gait trainers consist of 2 footplates positioned on 2 bars, 2 rockers, and 2 cranks, which provide the propulsive motion for the legs. The footplates generate the stance and swing phases in most instances with a symmetric motion.[41] Recent developments allow some degree of asymmetry in the trajectory selected for each leg. The main difference compared with exoskeletons with a treadmill is that the feet are always in contact with the moving platform, simulating the gait phases but not necessarily generating true swing and stance phases. The trajectories of the footplates, as well as the vertical and horizontal movements of the center of mass, are programmable. The end-effector design lends itself to gait retraining and stair climbing.[20] As a modality, this involves the least demand for the user to be able to initiate stepping motion and may result in greater variability in the knee and hip motion, as well as various levels of unweighing. Examples of end-effector devices include G-EO GTII, and Lokohelp.

A recent small randomized, prospective study compared 3 gait training techniques in persons with traumatic brain injury. It examined the impact of 3 different modes of locomotor therapy on gait velocity and spatiotemporal symmetry using an end-effector robot (G-EO), a robotic exoskeleton (Lokomat), and manually assisted partial-bodyweight–supported treadmill training in persons with traumatic brain injury. Subjects underwent 18 training sessions of 45 minutes duration each. Training elicited a statistically significant median increase in self-selected velocity for all groups compared with pretraining. Maximum velocity increased for the Lokomat but not the G-EO group. The mobility portion of the Stroke Impact Scale was significantly improved only for the Lokomat group. The study discussed the need of multiple staff and high physical demands to provide manual assistance for training. Staffing needed for therapy provision was the least for the Lokomat.[39]

In another comparative study, researchers took advantage of a clinical setup that placed a Lokomat and a G-EO next to each other with a 3-dimensional kinematic recording system. They obtained sequential data from subjects with spinal cord or traumatic brain injury diagnosis using the 2 systems and comparing that with bodyweight-supported manually assisted therapy on a treadmill. The data confirmed a more controlled and repetitive gait pattern when using a Lokomat with gait pattern that was most similar to that of overground walking. The G-EO provided a gait pattern that had more variability of motion for the hips and knees, with slightly reduced knee motion, and the gait pattern differed slightly from that observed during overground walking. Finally, the gait patterns achieved during manually assisted treadmill bodyweight-supported therapy were most variable with lack of symmetry of movement and timing. **Fig. 3** is a representative data set of the kinematics in a 32-year-old man with left spastic hemiparesis.[21]

Untethered Exoskeletons

Untethered exoskeletons are bilateral robots that incorporate actuators to move the patient's legs during the gait cycle, through a preprogrammed and near-normal gait

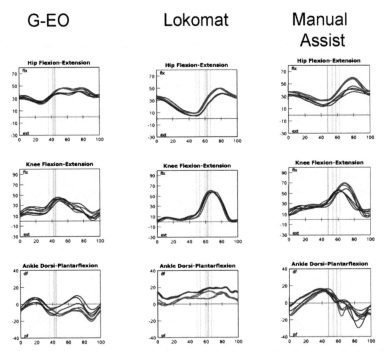

Fig. 3. A representative data set looking at the kinematics of a 32-year-old man with left spastic hemiparesis walking using 3 different gait training systems in a consecutive fashion. G-EO is an end-effector device, Lokomat a robotic exoskeleton device, manual assist is partial weightbearing treadmill training. Blue line = left limb, red line = right limb; data collected over multiple walking cycles with the CODA CX1 optoelectronic sensors.

cycle.[47] Their use usually requires upper limb aids to maintain balance (**Fig. 4**). They can also be divided into assistive and rehabilitative devices. The aim of assistive devices is to facilitate mobility in the home and community environments, whereas rehabilitative devices are intended to address the recovery of gait function in patients with neurologic injuries. In these devices, at least 2 joints are actuated (hip and knee) and, usually, 1 joint (ankle) is mechanically controlled. Robotic hip-knee-ankle-foot exoskeletal orthoses have become commercially available and may help patients to stand; walk; and, in some cases, climb steps. These devices also have applications beyond mobility; for example, exercise, amelioration of secondary complications related to lack of ambulation, and promotion of neuroplasticity.[48] Walking kinematics seem to vary widely both across individuals within a device,[49] as well as across devices.

Studies have shown the possibility of performing individual gait training in patients with a variety of pathologic conditions, including SCI, traumatic brain injury, stroke, and multiple sclerosis; the various CNS diagnoses for which exoskeletons are applicable were reviewed.[48] At present, for individuals with greater levels of impairment, wheelchairs remain the preferred mobility aid yet still fall considerably short compared with upright bipedal walking. Untethered exoskeletons hold much promise to fulfill this unmet need and have advanced substantially during the past decade as a viable option for both therapeutic and personal mobility purposes. A basic description of how the major exoskeleton devices work, a summary of key features, their known limitations, and a discussion of current and future clinical applicability have been comprehensively reviewed.[48]

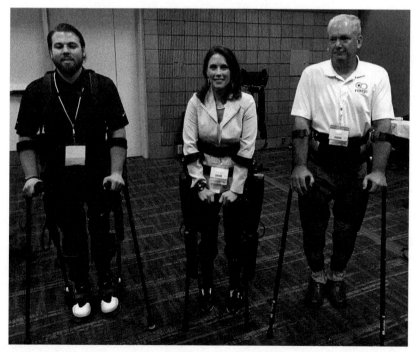

Fig. 4. Exoskeleton devices demonstrated at a recent educational event, from left to right: Ekso, ReWalk and Indego. (*Courtesy of* MossRehab with permission from ReWalk, Indego and Ekso.)

Patient-Guided Suspension Systems

Patient-guided suspension systems are nonanchored overground rolling frames that are inherently stable and provide a harness and/or trunk or pelvic support, with dynamic unweighing for some, while allowing the user freedom to initiate and carry out the walking movement. They include the Andago, SoloWalk (Gaittronics Inc. California USA),[50] KineAssist (Woodway, Wisconsin USA),[51] and WHERE-II (Korea).[52] Most have sensors and control algorithms to assist with propelling and maneuvering of the frame and adjusting and/or maintaining stable support.[53] This kind of robot allows the patients to walk overground and to explore the environment; patients are not confined to a fixed area. In some instances, the frame may be combined with untethered exoskeletons to offer the naturalistic independence of the latter with the safety of the former (**Fig. 5**).

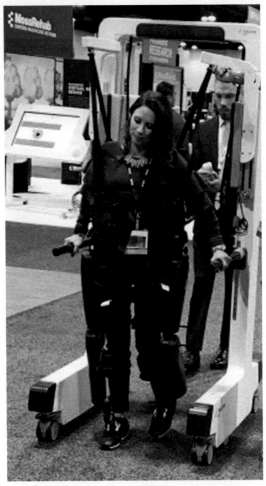

Fig. 5. Patient demonstrating the use of a ReWalk in combination with an Andago for training purposes. The combined systems may reduce the training staff needs compared with that of the exoskeleton alone, and provide an increased sense of security and stability during the initial training. (*Courtesy of* MossREhab with permission from ReWalk and Hocoma.)

DISCUSSION

The pace of development in all of these robotic technologies continues to increase, as well as to specialize. As an example, efforts are being directed toward niches such as improving the quality of the assisted gait patterns through the use of sensors and control algorithms.[40,54] The PubMed search criteria, (exoskeleton OR robot*) AND (walk* OR gait), revealed 2342 items with a timeline view showing the acceleration in recent years (**Fig. 6**).

Robotic technologies continue to be evaluated and show at least modest benefits across a variety of pathologic conditions; for example, children with cerebral palsy,[55] stroke,[25] SCI,[56] Parkinson disease, Brown-Sequard syndrome, and vascular dementia. It remains unclear, however, whether robot-assisted therapy is superior in certain clinical scenarios to conventional therapy. Finally, arguably, the most important outcome measure, quality of life, has begun to be studied as well.[57] In general, though there have been many reports of strong positive outcomes using robotics, the criteria and methodology for obtaining optimal benefits from robotics in the rehabilitation arena are still far from well-described[58]; however, there is also a growing effort to bring clarity to this field.[59] As an example, the ARTIC project that involves the formation of a diverse international panel of experts, a large combined patient cohort, standardized assessments, and a single robotic device (Lokomat).[58] Some investigators think that overground training has a higher potential for improving outcomes owing to biomechanics being more similar to natural gait.[53] There generally has been a deepened focus on understanding the active ingredients in robotic therapy along with a concerted effort to clarify relationships between dose and outcomes. More work is needed to define the therapeutic applications of these devices and further technical improvements are expected regarding device size; controls; and, for untethered devices, battery life and portability.

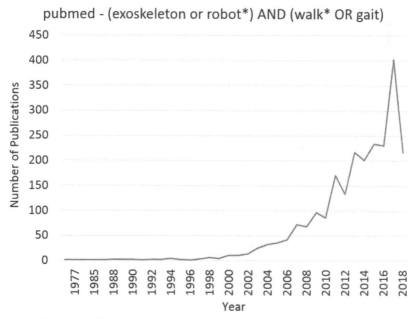

Fig. 6. Number of publications in robotics for gait rehabilitation by year over the past 4 decades. * To signify a wide search.

REFERENCES

1. Calabro RS, Cacciola A, Berte F, et al. Robotic gait rehabilitation and substitution devices in neurological disorders: where are we now? Neurol Sci 2016;37(4): 503–14.
2. Reinkensmeyer DJ, Emken JL, Cramer SC. Robotics, motor learning, and neurologic recovery. Annu Rev Biomed Eng 2004;6:497–525.
3. Esquenazi A, Lee S, Packel AT, et al. A randomized comparative study of manually assisted versus robotic-assisted body weight supported treadmill training in persons with a traumatic brain injury. PM R 2013;5(4):280–90.
4. Krakauer JW, Carmichael ST, Corbett D, et al. Getting neurorehabilitation right: what can be learned from animal models? Neurorehabil Neural Repair 2012; 26(8):923–31.
5. Kleim JA, Jones TA. Principles of experience-dependent neural plasticity: implications for rehabilitation after brain damage. J Speech Lang Hear Res 2008; 51(1):S225–39.
6. Murphy TH, Corbett D. Plasticity during stroke recovery: from synapse to behaviour. Nat Rev Neurosci 2009;10(12):861–72.
7. Dietz V. Neuronal plasticity after a human spinal cord injury: positive and negative effects. Exp Neurol 2012;235(1):110–5.
8. Edgerton VR, Tillakaratne NJ, Bigbee AJ, et al. Plasticity of the spinal neural circuitry after injury. Annu Rev Neurosci 2004;27:145–67.
9. Maier IC, Schwab ME. Sprouting, regeneration and circuit formation in the injured spinal cord: factors and activity. Philos Trans R Soc Lond B Biol Sci 2006; 361(1473):1611–34.
10. Dromerick AW, Lum PS, Hidler J. Activity-based therapies. NeuroRx 2006;3(4): 428–38.
11. Dietz V, Harkema SJ. Locomotor activity in spinal cord-injured persons. J Appl Physiol (1985) 2004;96(5):1954–60.
12. Kwakkel G, Wagenaar RC, Twisk JW, et al. Intensity of leg and arm training after primary middle-cerebral-artery stroke: a randomised trial. Lancet 1999; 354(9174):191–6.
13. Edgerton VR, de Leon RD, Tillakaratne N, et al. Use-dependent plasticity in spinal stepping and standing. Adv Neurol 1997;72:233–47.
14. Esquenazi A, Packel A. Robotic-assisted gait training and restoration. Am J Phys Med Rehabil 2012;91(11 Suppl 3):S217–27 [quiz: S228–31].
15. Iosa M, Morone G, Fusco A, et al. Seven capital devices for the future of stroke rehabilitation. Stroke Res Treat 2012;2012:187965.
16. Colombo G, Joerg M, Schreier R, et al. Treadmill training of paraplegic patients using a robotic orthosis. J Rehabil Res Dev 2000;37(6):693–700.
17. Veneman JF, Kruidhof R, Hekman EE, et al. Design and evaluation of the LOPES exoskeleton robot for interactive gait rehabilitation. IEEE Trans Neural Syst Rehabil Eng 2007;15(3):379–86.
18. Mantone J. Getting a leg up? Rehab patients get an assist from devices such as HealthSouth's AutoAmbulator, but the robots' clinical benefits are still in doubt. Mod Healthc 2006;36(7):58–60.
19. Hesse S, Uhlenbrock D, Werner C, et al. A mechanized gait trainer for restoring gait in nonambulatory subjects. Arch Phys Med Rehabil 2000;81(9):1158–61.
20. Hesse S, Waldner A, Tomelleri C. Innovative gait robot for the repetitive practice of floor walking and stair climbing up and down in stroke patients. J Neuroeng Rehabil 2010;7:30.

21. Esquenazi A, Maier IC, Schuler TA, et al. Clinical application of robotics and technology in the restoration of walking. In: D. R, V. D, editors. Neurorehabilitation technology. 2nd edition. Springer; 2016. p. 223–48.
22. Colombo G. The "Lokomat"-A driven ambulatory orthosis. Germany: dizinich Orthopadesche Technik 2000;6:178–81.
23. Allemand Y, Stauffer Y, Clavel R, et al. Design of a new lower extremity orthosis for overground gait training with the WalkTrainer. Paper presented at: 2009 IEEE International Conference on Rehabilitation Robotics. Kyoto, Japan, June 23–26, 2009.
24. Wang P, Low KH, Tow A, et al. Initial system evaluation of an overground rehabilitation gait training robot (NaTUre-gaits). Adv Robot 2011;25(15):1927–48.
25. Nam YG, Lee JW, Park JW, et al. Effects of electromechanical exoskeleton-assisted gait training on walking ability of stroke patients: a randomized controlled trial. Arch Phys Med Rehabil 2019;100(1):26–31.
26. Hornby TG, Campbell DD, Kahn JH, et al. Enhanced gait-related improvements after therapist-versus robotic-assisted locomotor training in subjects with chronic stroke: a randomized controlled study. Stroke 2008;39:1786–92.
27. Mayr A, Kofler M, Quirbach E, et al. Prospective, blinded, randomized crossover study of gait rehabilitation in stroke patients using the Lokomat gait orthosis. Neurorehabil Neural Repair 2007;21(4):307–14.
28. Hidler J, Nichols D, Pelliccio M, et al. Multicenter randomized clinical trial evaluating the effectiveness of the Lokomat in subacute stroke. Neurorehabil Neural Repair 2009;23(1):5–13.
29. Westlake KP, Patten C. Pilot study of Lokomat versus manual-assisted treadmill training for locomotor recovery post-stroke. J Neuroeng Rehabil 2009;6:18.
30. Vaney C, Gattlen B, Lugon-Moulin V, et al. Robotic-assisted step training (lokomat) not superior to equal intensity of over-ground rehabilitation in patients with multiple sclerosis. Neurorehabil Neural Repair 2012;26(3):212–21.
31. Alcobendas-Maestro M, Esclarin-Ruz A, Casado-Lopez RM, et al. Lokomat robotic-assisted versus overground training within 3 to 6 months of incomplete spinal cord lesion: randomized controlled trial. Neurorehabil Neural Repair 2012;26(9):1058–63.
32. Bonnyaud C, Pradon D, Boudarham J, et al. Effects of gait training using a robotic constraint (Lokomat(R)) on gait kinematics and kinetics in chronic stroke patients. J Rehabil Med 2014;46(2):132–8.
33. Bonnyaud C, Zory R, Boudarham J, et al. Effect of a robotic restraint gait training versus robotic conventional gait training on gait parameters in stroke patients. Exp Brain Res 2014;232(1):31–42.
34. Ucar DE, Paker N, Bugdayci D. Lokomat: a therapeutic chance for patients with chronic hemiplegia. NeuroRehabilitation 2014;34(3):447–53.
35. van Nunen MP, Gerrits KH, Konijnenbelt M, et al. Recovery of walking ability using a robotic device in subacute stroke patients: a randomized controlled study. Disabil Rehabil Assist Technol 2015;10(2):141–8.
36. Van Kammen K, Boonstra A, Reinders-Messelink H, et al. The combined effects of body weight support and gait speed on gait related muscle activity: a comparison between walking in the Lokomat exoskeleton and regular treadmill walking. PLoS One 2014;9(9):e107323.
37. Calabro RS, Reitano S, Leo A, et al. Can robot-assisted movement training (Lokomat) improve functional recovery and psychological well-being in chronic stroke? Promising findings from a case study. Funct Neurol 2014;29(2):139–41.

38. Calabro RS, De Luca R, Leo A, et al. Lokomat training in vascular dementia: motor improvement and beyond! Aging Clin Exp Res 2015;27(6):935–7.

39. Esquenazi A, Lee S, Wikoff A, et al. A comparison of locomotor therapy interventions: partial-body weight-supported treadmill, Lokomat, and G-EO training in people with traumatic brain injury. PM R 2017;9(9):839–46.

40. Wang D, Lee K. Sensor-guided gait synchronization for weight-support lower-extremity-exoskeleton. Paper presented at: 2016 IEEE International Conference on Advanced Intelligent Mechatronics (AIM). July 12–15, 2016.

41. Schmidt H, Werner C, Bernhardt R, et al. Gait rehabilitation machines based on programmable footplates. J Neuroeng Rehabil 2007;4:2.

42. Dzahir AM, Yamamoto S-I. Recent trends in lower-limb robotic rehabilitation orthosis: control scheme and strategy for pneumatic muscle actuated gait trainers. Robotics 2014;3(2):120–48.

43. Fisher S, Lucas L, Thrasher TA. Robot-assisted gait training for patients with hemiparesis due to stroke. Top Stroke Rehabil 2011;18(3):269–76.

44. Fleerkotte BM, Koopman B, Buurke JH, et al. The effect of impedance-controlled robotic gait training on walking ability and quality in individuals with chronic incomplete spinal cord injury: an explorative study. J Neuroeng Rehabil 2014; 11:26.

45. Brutsch K, Koenig A, Zimmerli L, et al. Virtual reality for enhancement of robot-assisted gait training in children with central gait disorders. J Rehabil Med 2011;43(6):493–9.

46. Labruyere R, Gerber CN, Birrer-Brutsch K, et al. Requirements for and impact of a serious game for neuro-pediatric robot-assisted gait training. Res Dev Disabil 2013;34(11):3906–15.

47. Molteni F, Gasperini G, Gaffuri M, et al. Wearable robotic exoskeleton for overground gait training in sub-acute and chronic hemiparetic stroke patients: preliminary results. Eur J Phys Rehabil Med 2017;53(5):676–84.

48. Esquenazi A, Talaty M, Jayaraman A. Powered exoskeletons for walking assistance in persons with central nervous system injuries: a narrative review. PM R 2017;9(1):46–62.

49. Talaty M, Esquenazi A, Briceno JE. Differentiating ability in users of the ReWalk(TM) powered exoskeleton: an analysis of walking kinematics. IEEE Int Conf Rehabil Robot 2013;2013:6650469.

50. McCormick A, Alazem H, Morbi A, et al. Power Walker helps a child with cerebral palsy. 3rd International Conference on Control, Dynamic Systems, and Robotics. Ottawa, Canada, May 9–10, 2016.

51. Patton J, Brown DA, Peshkin M, et al. KineAssist: design and development of a robotic overground gait and balance therapy device. Top Stroke Rehabil 2008; 15(2):131–9.

52. Seo KH, Lee JJ. The development of two mobile gait rehabilitation systems. IEEE Trans Neural Syst Rehabil Eng 2009;17(2):156–66.

53. Alias NA, Huq MS, Ibrahim BSKK, et al. The efficacy of state of the art overground gait rehabilitation robotics: a bird's eye view. Procedia Comput Sci 2017;105: 365–70.

54. Chen QA-O, Cheng HA-O, Yue C, et al. Dynamic balance gait for walking assistance exoskeleton. Appl Bionics Biomech 2018;2018:7847014.

55. Carvalho I, Pinto SM, Chagas DDV, et al. Robotic gait training for individuals with cerebral palsy: a systematic review and meta-analysis. Arch Phys Med Rehabil 2017;98(11):2332–44.

56. Esquenazi A, Talaty M, Packel A, et al. The ReWalk powered exoskeleton to restore ambulatory function to individuals with thoracic-level motor-complete spinal cord injury. Am J Phys Med Rehabil 2012;91(11):911–21.
57. EA-Ohoo Yilmaz, Schmidt CK, Mayadev A, et al. Does treadmill training with hybrid assistive limb (HAL) impact the quality of life? A first case series in the United States. Disabil Rehabil Assist Technol 2018;1–5. https://doi.org/10.1080/17483107.2018.1493751.
58. van Hedel HJA, Severini G, Scarton A, et al. Advanced Robotic Therapy Integrated Centers (ARTIC): an international collaboration facilitating the application of rehabilitation technologies. J Neuroeng Rehabil 2018;15(1):30.
59. Bayon C, Martin-Lorenzo T, Moral-Saiz B, et al. A robot-based gait training therapy for pediatric population with cerebral palsy: goal setting, proposal and preliminary clinical implementation. J Neuroeng Rehabil 2018;15(1):69.

Validity and Reliability of the Kinect for Assessment of Standardized Transitional Movements and Balance

Systematic Review and Translation into Practice

Urška Puh, PT, PhD[a], Brittany Hoehlein, SDPT[b],
Judith E. Deutsch, PT, PhD[b,*]

KEYWORDS

• Kinect • Validity • Reliability • Standardized tests • Balance

KEY POINTS

• The Kinect versions 1 and 2 have shown criterion, construct, concurrent, and discriminant validity for healthy adults and persons with the following health conditions: multiple sclerosis, Parkinson disease, stroke, frail older adults, low back pain.
• The reliability of the Kinect cameras versions 1 and 2 has been tested less than validity.
• Modest validity and reliability of the Kinect versions 1 and 2 cameras have been shown for the Five Times Sit to Stand, Timed Up and Go, the Functional Reach Test, and stepping activities.
• Modest validity and reliability have been shown for single-limb and double-limb balance testing with Kinect cameras versions 1 and 2 with decreased reliability during more complex measurements, such as standing on foam.
• Translation of the standardized assessments into practice is limited by access to software.

INTRODUCTION

Game consoles such as the Nintendo Wii Balance Board (WBB) and the Microsoft Kinect have force and motion sensors originally designed to sense movement for interactive games. However, they can also be used to measure kinematics and

Disclosure: The authors have nothing to disclose.
[a] Department of Physiotherapy, Faculty of Health Sciences, University of Ljubljana, Zdravstvena pot 5, Ljubljana 1000, Slovenia; [b] Rivers Lab, Department of Rehabilitation and Movement Science, School of Health Professions, Rutgers University, 65 Bergen Street, Newark, NJ 07101, USA
* Corresponding author.
E-mail address: deutsch@shp.rutgers.edu

Phys Med Rehabil Clin N Am 30 (2019) 399–422
https://doi.org/10.1016/j.pmr.2018.12.006
1047-9651/19/© 2018 Elsevier Inc. All rights reserved.

kinetics of movement. Their low cost and portability have made them desirable alternatives to laboratory-based tools. Open access as development platforms with documentation of how to acquire the data provided online, ease of implementation,[1,2] and development of customized software for use in the WBB and both Kinect versions as assessment tools have recently increased dramatically. Consequently, there have been several studies investigating the validity and reliability of these off-the-shelf tools. A review of these systems in orthopedics by Ruff and colleagues[3] concluded that commercially available gaming systems have the potential to serve as low cost but accurate and reliable clinical assessment tools. However, care must be taken in evaluating the reliability, accuracy, sensitivity, and specificity of these devices before their use in clinical applications.[3]

The WBB is a force sensor used to measure center of pressure, which is a useful metric for balance assessments. A recently published systematic review[2] indicated that, although the WBB has limitations as a measurement tool, it can provide data for static standing that are concurrently valid with typical commercial force platforms and have reliability similar to force platforms' computerized posturography.

The Kinect sensor relies on vision-based body tracking, which uses computer vison to track human motion in 3 dimensions. The sensor comprises a red, green, and blue camera and a depth-sensing camera to provide data, which are then processed with advanced computer algorithms. These algorithms enable the position and orientation of body joints to be determined.[1,4] Microsoft released a beta version of the Kinect software development kit for Kinect 360 (version 1; V1) in 2011, and Kinect One (version 2; V2) was released in 2014, facilitating the development of software for purposes other than recreation. Compared with other commercially available depth sensors, such as the Leap sensor and Intel Creative camera, the Kinect is superior at measuring lower limb and full-body motion.[1,5] Further, the reliability of Kinect when analyzing planar motions has been shown to be similar to three-dimensional (3D) marker-based motion analysis (3DMA) systems.[1] A proposed advantage of using the Kinect as a clinical assessment tool is that it is a markerless motion capture system[6] compared with laboratory 3DMA systems, increasing its feasibility for use in investigating these parameters in everyday clinical practice.

In contrast with the WBB, vison-based body tracking with Kinect enables not only assessment of static or dynamic balance[7,8] but also measurement of variety of whole-body,[9–11] upper-limb,[12–14] and functional movements, as well as long-term movement monitoring (eg, in intensive care unit),[15] at home[16,17] or in the workplace.[18] The validity of the Kinect to measure temporal and spatial measures of gait was reviewed by Springer and Yogev Seligman.[19] The review included studies of gait under different conditions, such as walking on the treadmill, stepping in place,[20] and Timed Up and Go (TUG) test,[9] as well as collection of data with 4 Kinect sensors.[21] Despite the heterogeneity of the review, the investigators concluded that Kinect is valid for some temporal and displacement parameters. However, the kinematic parameters showed poor validity and large errors.[19]

Although the Kinect may have some limitations in its validity for measuring translation movement such as gait, it may be a useful tool to quantify transitional movements and balance tasks. The assessment of these tasks requires less space than gait and they are also commonly assessed in physical therapy practice. Therefore, this systematic review evaluates the validity and reliability of the Kinect in measuring transitional movements, stepping, and static and dynamic balance and determines whether the tests could be translated and implemented in practice.

METHODS

Relevant publications were identified by searching the electronic databases PubMed, EBSCO*host*/Cumulative Index of Nursing and Allied Health Literature (CINAHL with Full Text), and IEEE (Institute of Electrical and Electronics Engineers) Xplore Digital Library using a search string in PubMed (**Table 1**). The databases were searched by indexing terms (MeSH) and free-text terms used with synonyms and related terms in the title or abstract. The Boolean operator AND linked the game console to the tests, which were summed using the Boolean operator OR (eg: "kinect" and "sit to stand" or "timed up and go" or "stepping" or "balance"). This search strategy was adapted for CINAHL and IEEE. The full search strategy can be obtained from the corresponding author. All databases were last searched on June 11, 2018. In addition, references of the included articles and published relevant reviews were reviewed. Two review authors (U.P., B.H.) independently screened the titles and abstracts and assessed publications in full text for eligibility. In case of disagreement between the two reviewers, the third reviewer (J.D.) reconciled these differences.

The search was restricted to the English language. Review articles, study protocols, conference abstracts and posters, and theses were not included in the review. Studies were included if validity or reliability of spatiotemporal parameters and/or kinematics measured with a single Kinect sensor were analyzed as an existing or potential clinical test of the following tasks:

- Transitional movement (eg, sit to stand)
- Stepping behavior (eg, step test, marching in place)
- Standardized balance tasks in standing

Studies were excluded if the Kinect sensor was used: (1) for measurement of reaction time, (2) solely to analyze sport-related activities (eg, squats, jumps, hops, lunges, martial arts), (3) to monitor general movement (eg, continuous in-home or workplace monitoring), (4) for assessment during a game, and (5) in combination with other devices (eg, WBB, perturbation system). In addition, studies were excluded if absence of any conventional report of validity or reliability was identified during data extraction.

Data were extracted by using a predetermined table with the following categories: subjects' characteristics, Kinect version and settings, type and results for validity, and

Table 1 Search strategy PubMed	
#1	Search ((kinect[Title/Abstract] OR xbox[Title/Abstract])) AND Sit to stand [Title/Abstract]
#2	Search ((kinect[Title/Abstract] OR xbox[Title/Abstract]) AND (TUG[Title/Abstract] OR timed up[Title/Abstract] OR get up[Title/Abstract]))
#3	Search (((kinect[Title/Abstract] OR xbox[Title/Abstract])) AND (step*[Title/Abstract] OR walking on the spot[Title/Abstract] OR marching in place [Title/Abstract]))
#4	Search (((((kinect[Title/Abstract] OR xbox[Title/Abstract])) AND (balance [Title/Abstract] OR postural control[Title/Abstract] OR posturography [Title/Abstract] OR sway[Title/Abstract] OR stability[Title/Abstract] OR balance, postural[Mesh]))))
#5	Search #1 OR #2 OR#3 OR #4

type and results for reliability. Results were extracted for each Kinect parameter or in ranges for the groups of parameters. Additional details of the test conditions (eg, visual, foam, step width) were extracted and represented in figures.

The quality of the study's methodology was rated using criteria and a 3-point scale adapted from the consensus-based, standards for the selection of health measurement instruments (COSMIN) checklist.[22] Studies were rated a high quality (by 2 raters U.P., J.D.) if they had (1) an adequate sample size (n $\geq$10) based on the use of an objective measure of motion, (2) an accurate execution of the standardized tests, (3) a reproducible description of methodology, and (4) an analysis of both validity and reliability. They were rated as medium-quality studies if they had 3 of the 4 characteristics of the high-quality studies, and as low quality if they had 2 or fewer of the characteristics of the high-quality studies.

Validity and reliability data were rated for the strength of statistical results based on published criteria.[23,24] For criterion validity (compared with gold standard), and concurrent validity (compared with related clinical tests) and reliability, intraclass correlation coefficients (ICCs), Pearson correlation coefficients (r), or cross-correlation coefficients were extracted. Strength of the validity and reliability were rated as follows: a coefficient less than 0.5 indicated poor, from 0.5 to 0.75 indicated moderate, from 0.75 to 0.9 indicated good, and values more than 0.90 indicated excellent reliability or validity.[23,24] When correlation coefficients were not reported, Bland-Altman plots using the limits of 95% agreement were substituted instead. For construct validity, Pearson (r) or Spearman correlation coefficients (ρ) were extracted. Values less than 0.25 indicated little or no relationship, between 0.25 and 0.50 indicated fair, between 0.50 and 0.75 indicated moderate to good, and values greater than 0.75 indicated good to excellent relationships.[23] Discriminant validity was confirmed if a statistically significant difference was reported to document differences between the known groups.[23]

The investigators of the studies identified as high or medium quality were contacted by email for clarification of their methods and a request for reliability testing if it was not reported. At most, 3 email queries were sent, and in 1 instance a phone call was required to reach the investigators. Once it was determined that the article had both reported validity and reliability, and it was of sufficient quality, the investigators were queried about whether their software was available and whether they were willing to share it. This final step was relevant for assessing the likelihood of translation of the findings into practice. Articles were recommended for clinical practice if the quality was high and the strength of the criterion and concurrent validity and reliability statistics was excellent or good.

RESULTS

The search results are presented in the preferred reporting items for systematic reviews and meta-analyses (PRISMA) format in **Fig. 1**. During data extraction, 2 studies[25,26] were excluded because criterion validity was not reported using a standard method. The remaining 21 research articles, published from 2012 to 2018, were included in the analysis and qualitative synthesis. Results are presented in **Tables 2–6**. Twenty-one studies assessed validity and 10 investigated reliability.[7–9,27–32] Criterion validity was assessed in 12 studies.[7,8,20,27,30,32–38] In 6 studies, concurrent validity of the Kinect measurements was compared with results of the corresponding clinical test[9,28,29,39,40] or with measurements with the WBB.[41] Discriminant validity was assessed in 7 studies[28,29,31,32,39,42,43] and construct validity in 5.[28,29,31,41,43]

The Kinect sensor V1 was used in 10 studies,[7–9,20,28–30,35,36,40] and V2 in 11 studies.[27,31–34,37–39,41–43] Different 3DMA systems and/or force plates were used as

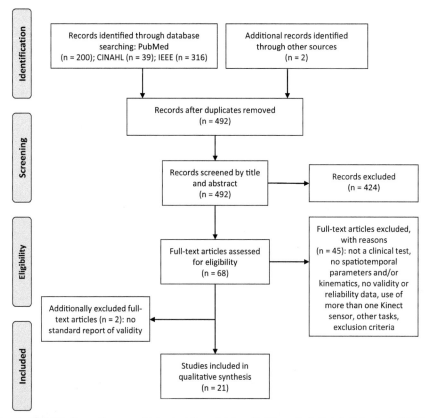

Fig. 1. PRISMA flow diagram. (*Adapted from* Moher D, Liberati A, Tetzlaff J, et al, PRISMA Group. Reprint–preferred reporting items for systematic reviews and meta-analyses: the PRISMA statement. Phys Ther 2009;89(9):873–80; with permission.)

the criterion reference: Vicon,[7,8,20,27,33] Qualisys AB,[34] Optotrack,[30,35] SMART-DX,[37,38] BTS-Elite with Kistler force plate,[32] and nonspecified force plate.[8,36]

Most studies (N = 14) included only healthy subjects. In 5 studies, participants had different health conditions: inpatient frail older adults,[39] Parkinson disease,[20] stroke,[9] multiple sclerosis (MS),[31] and low back pain.[32] In 2 studies with older adults,[28,29] the health condition of subjects was not reported; the investigators stated that individuals with severe or medically unstable health conditions were excluded from participation. Sample sizes varied from 3[34] to 442[29] participants. In total, there were 1188 participants, including 466 healthy subjects (young adults, n = 186; young and middle-aged adults, n = 178; master athletes, n = 30; older adults, n = 72), 186 patients, and 536 older adults with no specific defined health condition.

Studies that measured transitional movement included the Five Times Sit to Stand (5TSTS) test,[20,27,28,34,42,43] (see **Table 2**), the TUG test[9,34,39] (see **Table 3**), and measurements of 4 different stepping patterns[20,27,34] (see **Table 4**). Balance was reported for 4 dynamic[7,29,35,37] and 3 static balance tests under different test conditions[7,8,27,30–33,36,40–43] (see **Table 5** for the Kinect V1 and **Table 6** for the Kinect V2). The number of reported Kinect parameters per test varied from 1[33,35,36,40,41] to 35.[34]

Table 2
Measurement of Five Times Sit to Stand test using Kinect

Study	Subjects (n)	Kinect Version; Orientation and Distance	Validity (Comparison)	Reliability			Quality/ Recommend/ Available
Ejupi et al,[28] 2016	Healthy OA: Validity (94); reliability supervised (18), unsupervised (13)	V1 0.8 m height, 2 m in front of the subject	**Concurrent** (5 times STS clinical): TT r = 0.99, mean STS velocity r = −0.59 **Construct** (strength): TT r = −0.32, mean STS velocity r = 0.53; (balance): TT r = 0.23, mean STS velocity r = −0.25; (reaction time): mean STS velocity r = −0.32 **Discriminant** (fallers vs nonfallers): mean STS velocity ES d = 0.67	Test-retest (40 ± 20 d) laboratory vs home			H Y: total time, STS velocity N: unable to contact author
					Home supervised	Home unsupervised	
				TT	r = 0.83	0.92	
				STS velocity	r = 0.70	0.93	
Otte et al,[27] 2016	YA (19)	V2 1.4 m height (vertical angle of −8°), 2.5 m in front of the subject	**Criterion** (3DMA): time ICC = 0.92–0.95, AP trunk displ ICC = 0.93–0.99, ML trunk displ ICC = 0.73–0.78	Within session (5 rep)			H Y: up- and down-time, AP trunk displacement Y: Motognosis for research
					Kinect	3DMA	
				Time	ICC = 0.55–0.72	0.62–0.77	
				AP trunk displ	ICC = 0.73–0.81	0.79–0.82	
				ML trunk displ	ICC = 0.49–0.56	0.33–0.43	
Galna et al,[20] 2014	YA (10) PD (9)	V1 1 m height (lens perpendicular to the floor), 3 m in front of the subject	**Criterion** (3DMA): TT: YA ICC = 0.96, PD ICC = 0.99; vertical head displ: YA ICC = 0.99, PD ICC = 0.98	—			M/N Y: Microsoft SDK for research

Study	Groups	Setup	Results	Recommendation
Leightley and Yap,[42] 2018	YA (15) Healthy OA (10) MA (15)	V2 0.7 m height, 2 m in front of the subject	Discriminant (YA, MA, MA): TT did not differ between groups, stand time (YA/MA), AP CoM displ stand (YA/OA), ML CoM displ sit (YA/OA and OA/MA), sit trunk angle (YA/OA; YA/MA), sit velocity (YA/MA)	M/N Y: for research
Leightley et al,[43] 2017	YA (15) Healthy OA (13) MA runners (15)	V2 0.7 m height, 2 m in front of the subject	Construct (1LST EC with Kinect): AP CoM displ r = −0.33, ML CoM displ r = −0.42 Discriminant (YA, OA, MA): TT no difference between groups, AP CoM displ (YA/OA and YA/MA)	M/N Y: for research
Napoli et l,[34] 2017	YA (3)	V2 2–4 m in front of the subject	Criterion (3DMA): Joint displacements AP CCC = 0.41–0.99 Vertical CCC = 0.39–0.99 ML CCC = 0.34–0.99 Joint angles r = 0.25–0.98	L/N

Abbreviations: </=/>, lower/equal/higher than reliability of the gold standard; 3DMA, 3D motion analysis system; AP/ML, anteroposterior/mediolateral movement plane; CCC, cross-correlation coefficient; CoM, center of body mass; displ, displacement; ES, effect size; H/M/L, study of high/medium/low quality; ICC, intraclass correlation coefficient; MA, master athletes; OA, older adults; PD, patients with Parkinson disease; r, Pearson correlation coefficient; SDK, software development kit; STS, sit to stand; TT, total time; V1, Kinect 360; V2, Kinect One; Y/N, yes/no recommendation/available; YA, young adults.

Table 3
Measurement of timed up and go using kinect

Study	Subjects (n)	Kinect Version; Orientation and Distance	Validity (Comparison)	Reliability		Quality/ Recommend/ Available
				Test-Retest (7 d)		
Vernon et al,[9] 2015	Stroke (30)	V1 Off-center 0.8 m, 3 m from the starting point	**Concurrent** (TUG clinical) TT ρ = 0.99	TT Turning time Trunk flex angle Flex angle velocity Step and stride length, gait speed	ICC = 0.99 ICC = 0.99 ICC = 0.73 ICC = 0.93 ICC = 0.94–0.98	H Y: TT Y: outdated not supported
Dubois et al,[39] 2018	Inpatient frail OA (37)	V2 4 m from the walking pathway, sagittal view	**Concurrent** (TUG clinical; 2 clinicians): TT ICC = 0.99 **Discriminant** (low vs high risk of fall) for 21 spatial and temporal parameters at a 13.5 s cutoff	—		M/N/N: unable to contact
Napoli et al,[34] 2017	YA (3)	V2 2–4 m in front of the subject	**Criterion** (3DMA): Joint displacements AP CCC = 0.90–0.99, vertical CCC = 0.07–0.98, ML CCC = 0.64–0.97; Joint angles CCC = 0.11–1	—		L/N/N

Height of the camera was not provided.
Abbreviations: 3DMA, 3D motion analysis system; AP/ML, anteroposterior/mediolateral movement plane; CCC, cross-correlation coefficient; flex, flexion; H/M/L, study of high/medium/low quality; ICC, intraclass correlation coefficient; OA, older adults; TT, total time; TUG, timed up and go test; V1, Kinect 360; V2, Kinect One; Y/N, yes/no recommendation/available; YA, young adults; ρ, Spearman correlation coefficient.

Table 4
Measurement of stepping using Kinect

Study	Subjects (n)	Task	Kinect Version; Orientation and Distance	Validity (Comparison)	Reliability		Quality/ Recommend/ Available
Otte et al,[27] 2016	YA (19)	Stepping in place	V2 1.4 m height (vertical angle of −8°), 2.5 m in front of the subject	**Criterion (3DMA):** Cadence ICC = 1, AP-vertical knee displ ICC = 0.10–0.12	Within Session (3 Rep) Kinect 3DMA Cadence ICC = 0.96–0.98 0.96–0.98 AP-vertical ICC = 0.86–0.93 0.91–0.93 knee displ		H Y: Cadence Y: Motognosis for research
Galna et al,[20] 2014	YA (10), PD (9)	Stepping in place, forward stepping, side stepping	V1 1 m height (lens perpendicular to the floor), 3 m in front of the subject	**Criterion (3DMA):** Stepping in place time/rep: YA and PD ICC = 0.97–0.99, vertical knee displ: YA ICC = 0.78, PD ICC = 0.71 Forward stepping time/rep: YA and PD ICC = 0.98, Hip flex angle: YA ICC = 0.74, PD ICC = 0.78 Side stepping time/rep: YA and PD ICC = 0.94–0.99 Hip abd angle: YA and PD ICC = 0.78–0.88	—		M/N Y: Microsoft software development kit
Napoli et al,[34] 2017	YA (3)	Marching in place	V2 2–4 m in front of the subject	**Criterion (3DMA):** Joint displacements AP CCC = 0.53–0.99, vertical CCC = 0.23–0.99, ML CCC = 0.74–0.99; Joint angles CCC = 0.13–0.95	—		L/N

Abbreviations: 3DMA, 3D motion analysis system; abd, abduction; AP/ML, anteroposterior/mediolateral movement plane; CCC, cross-correlation coefficient; flex, flexion; H/M/L, study of high/medium/low quality; ICC, intraclass correlation coefficient; PD, patients with Parkinson's disease ; rep, repetition, V1, Kinect 360; V2, Kinect One; Y/N, yes/no recommendation/available; YA, young adults.

Table 5
Measurement of dynamic and static balance in standing position using Kinect version 1

Study	Test	Subjects (n)	Kinect Orientation and Distance	Validity (Comparison)	Reliability	Quality/Recommend/Available
Clark et al,[7] 2012	FRT, lateral reach, 1LST EC	YA (20)	2.5 m in front of the subject	Criterion (3DMA): FRT: Reach distance r = 0.95, sternum displ r = 0.90, trunk flex angle r = 0.98; Lateral reach: Reach distance r = 0.84, sternum displ r = 0.94, Trunk lat flex angle r = 0.93; 1LST: Ankle-, knee displ r = 0.92–0.97, AP-, ML pelvis and sternum displ, trunk angles r = 0.98–0.99	Within Session (2 Rep): Kinect / 3DMA — FRT; Lateral Reach: Reach distance ICC = 0.81–0.89 / 0.77–0.89; Sternum displ, trunk lat flex angle ICC = 0.73 / 0.89, ICC = 0.87–0.89 / 0.86; 1LST: Ankle, knee displ ICC = 0.64–0.71 / 0.77–0.81; AP pelvis and sternum displ ICC = 0.26–0.46 / 0.25–0.36; ML pelvis and sternum displ ICC = 0.56–0.70 / 0.68; Trunk angles ICC = 0.54–0.69 / 0.45–0.66	H; Y: FRT Lateral reach: sternum displ, lat trunk flex angle; Y: outdated
Hsiao et al,[29] 2018	FRT	OA: <75 y (278), ≥75 y (164)	Shoulder height, at right side and 1.8 m from the subject	Concurrent (FRT clinical): Reach distance r = 0.72, shoulder velocity at halfway time r = 0.24; Construct (posturography): velocity at halfway time r = −0.26; Discriminant (<75 vs ≥ 75 y): significant for reach distance	Within Session (2 Rep): Reach distance ICC = 0.82; Velocity at halfway time ICC = 0.77	H; Y: reach distance; N: Unable to contact
Yeung et al,[8] 2014	2LST: EO, EC, EOf, ECf	YA (10)	1 m height, 3 m from the subject	Criterion 3DMA / Force plate: AP CoM displ r = 0.94–0.95 / 0.76–0.90; ML CoM displ r = 0.93–0.99 / 0.88–0.95	Within Session (2 Rep): Kinect / 3DMA / Force plate: AP CoM displ ICC = 0.37–0.81 / 0.47–0.70 / 0.18–0.58; ML CoM displ ICC = 0.16–0.55 / 0.25–0.57 / 0.12–0.61	H/N; N: MS SDK and CoM share with researchers

Study	Population	Test	Distance	Criterion	Within Session (2 Rep) Kinect	3DMA	M/ Y/N
Yang et al,[30] 2014	YA (9)	2LST: feet apart, feet together; EO 1LST: EO	2.5 m from the subject	**Criterion (3DMA):** 2LST H CoM displ RMS ICC = 0.95–0.98, H CoM SVx ICC = 0.93–0.96 1LST H CoM displ RMS ICC = 0.95–0.96, H CoM SVx ICC = 0.88–0.96	2LST H CoM displ RMS ICC = 0.75–0.94 H CoM SVx ICC = 0.92–0.96 1LST H CoM displ RMS ICC = 0.76 H CoM SVx ICC = 0.87	0.83–0.85 0.88–0.93 0.76 0.84	M/ Y: 1LST, 2LST N: unable to contact
Galen et al,[35] 2015 FRT interactive	YA (20)		0.87 m height, offset in forward direction 0.75 from lateral line, at 2.0, 2.5, and 3.0 m to the left of the FRT line	**Criterion (3DMA):** Reach distance for 3 Kinect placements: 2.0 m ICC = 0.62, 2.5 m ICC = 0.73, 3.0 m ICC = 0.71	No reliability available at the time of the systematic review because their development is ongoing		M/N/N
Chakravarty et al,[36] 2016	1LST: EO	HA (35)	1.37 m height, 2.1–2.4 m from the subject	**Criterion (force plate):** Test duration 97% points were contained in the 95% CI on Bland and Altman plot			M/N/ N: unable to contact
Choi et al,[40] 2016	1LST: EO	YA (5)	2 m in front of the subject	**Concurrent (1LST clinical):** Test duration: absolute error = 0.37 s			L/N

Abbreviations: 1LST, single-leg stance test; 2LST, double-leg stance test; 3DMA, 3D motion analysis system; AP/ML/H, anteroposterior/mediolateral/horizontal movement plane; CI, confidence interval; CoM, center of body mass; displ, displacement; EC, eyes closed; EO, eyes open; flex, flexion; f, foam; FRT, functional reach test; HA, healthy adults (young and middle aged); H/M/L, study of high/ medium/low quality; ICC, intraclass correlation coefficient; lat, lateral; OA, older adults; RMS, root mean square; r, Pearson's correlation coefficient; SVx, mean sway velocity; Y/N, yes/no recommen- dation/available; YA, young adults.

Table 6
Measurement of dynamic and static balance in standing position using Kinect version 2

Study	Test	Subjects (n)	Kinect Orientation and Distance	Validity (Comparison)	Reliability		Quality/Recommend/Available
Clark et al,[33] 2015	FRT, lateral reach, limits of stability, 2LST: EO EC, 1LST: EO, EC	YA (30)	2.5 m in front of the subject	**Criterion (3DMA):** <u>FRT</u> Trunk flex angle r = 0.93 <u>Lateral reach</u> Trunk lat flex angle r = 0.92 <u>Limits of stability</u> Trunk flex and lat flex angles r = 0.83–0.98 <u>2LST</u> AP sternum, pelvis, displ and path length r = 0.81–0.94, ML sternum, pelvis, displ and path length r = 0.06–0.44 <u>1LST</u> AP sternum, pelvis, displ and path length r = 0.87–0.95, ML sternum, pelvis, displ and path length r = 0.49–0.82	**Test Retest (7 ± 2 d)** Kinect *FRT* ICC = 0.72 *Lateral reach* ICC = 0.85 *Limits of stability* ICC = 0.88–0.91 *2LST* AP displ and path length ICC = 0.80–0.90 ML displ and path length ICC = 0.03–0.79 *1LST* AP displ and path length ICC = 0.18–0.71 ML displ and path length ICC = 0.08–0.90	3DMA 0.81 0.82 0.85–0.88 0.69–0.94 0.44–0.92 0.03–0.79 0.30–0.93	H Y: FRT Lateral reach Limits of stability 2LST: AP sternum, pelvis displ, path length N: not supported
Otte et al,[27] 2016	2LST: EO and EC (in 1 test)	YA (19)	1.4 m height (vertical angle of −8°), 2.5 m in front of the subject	**Criterion (3DMA):** AP, 3D CoM displ angle, CoM Sωx ICC = 0.92–0.97 ML CoM displ angle ICC = 0.81	**Within Session (5 Rep)** Kinect — AP, ML, 3D CoM displ angles ICC = 0.41–0.47 AP, ML- 3D CoM Sωx ICC = 0.75–0.82	3DMA 0.36–0.43 0.77–0.84	H Y: 2LST AP, ML and 3D CoM sway Y: for research

Study	Test conditions	Sample	Setup	Results	Reliability (Within Session [3 Rep] / Test-retest)	H
Behrens et al,[31] 2016	2LST feet apart, feet together; Tandem: EO, EC	Validity: HA (59), MS (90); Reliability: HA (36), MS (18)	1.4 m height, 2.3 m in front of the subject (mean distance)	**Construct** relative to clinical disability scales (EDSS, timed 25-foot walk, MSWS-12): 2LST EC: ↑ 3D CoM S_{oX} was associated with ↓ walking speed, ↓ EDSS scores (mainly cerebellar functional system score), and reflected self-reported walking disability. **Discriminant** (HA, MS): MS significantly higher AP, ML, 3D CoM S_{oX} in all test conditions than HA	**Within Session (3 Rep)** — HA / MS: 2LST — AP S_{oX} ICC = 0.55–0.75 / 0.88–0.97; ML S_{oX} ICC = 0.71–0.85 / 0.91–0.94; 3D S_{oX} ICC = 0.65–0.80 / 0.94–0.98. Tandem — AP S_{oX} ICC = 0.56–0.67 / 0.82–0.88; ML S_{oX} ICC = 0.55–0.65 / 0.68–0.81; 3D S_{oX} ICC = 0.54–0.71 / 0.76–0.84	H — Y: 2LST 3D CoM sway velocity for HA and MS; Y: for research
Grooten et al,[32] 2018	2LST: EO, 1LST: EO	Criterion: HA (30); Discriminant: HA (17), LBP (20); Reliability: HA (37)	0.82–0.86 m height, 3m in front of subject	**Criterion** (3DMA with force plate): 2LST — CoM sway area ICC = 0.35; AP, ML CoM SV_{max} ICC = 0.04. 1LST — CoM sway area ICC = 0.11–0.42, AP, ML CoM SV_{max} ICC = 0.01–0.30. **Discriminant** (HA, LBP): significant difference only for AP CoM SV_{max} at 1LST with the right leg	**Test-retest (7 ± 1 d)**: 2LST ICC = 0.01–0.12; 1LST ICC = 0.05–0.23	H/N
Leightley et al,[43] 2017	2LST: EO, Semitandem: EO, Tandem: EO, 1LST: EO, EC	YA (15), Healthy OA (13), MA runners (15)	0.7 m height, 2 m in front of the subject	**Construct** (FTSTS with Kinect): 1LST EC: see **Table 2**. **Discriminant** (YA, OA, MA): 2LST — ML CoM displ (YA/OA, OA/MA); Semitandem and Tandem — ML, AP CoM displ (YA/OA, OA/MA); 1LST — EO: ML, AP CoM displ (YA/OA); EC: test duration (YA/OA/MA); ML, AP CoM displ (YA/OA, YA/MA)	—	M/N — Y: available on GitHub. https://leightley.com/recording-kinect-one-streams-using-c/https://github.com/DrDanL/KinectRecorder

(continued on next page)

Table 6
(continued)

Study	Test	Subjects (n)	Kinect Orientation and Distance	Validity (Comparison)	Reliability	Quality/Recommend/Available
Eltoukhy et al,[38] 2018	1LST: EO, EC	YA (10) Healthy OA (10)	Waist height, 2.5 m in front of the subject	Criterion (3DMA) $\quad$ YA $\quad$ OA Test duration $\quad$ ICC = 1 $\quad$ 0.99 AP, ML CoM displ $\;$ ICC = 0.97–0.99 $\;$ 0.97–1 AP, ML SVx $\quad$ ICC = 0.96–0.99 $\;$ 0.91–0.99 H average $\quad$ ICC = 0.89–0.99 $\;$ 0.97–1 CoM displ	—	M/N
Eltoukhy et al,[37] 2017	YBT	YA (10)	0.75 m height, 2.5 m in front of the subject	**Criterion (3DMA):** All reach distances ICC = 0.99 Anterior direction joint angles $\quad$ ICC = 0.73–0.99 Posteromedial direction joint angles $\quad$ ICC = 0.88–0.99 Posterolateral direction joint angles $\quad$ ICC = 0.00–0.99	—	M/N
Mazumder et al,[41] 2017	1LST: EO	Concurrent: YA (10) Construct: Healthy OA: 65–69 y (15), 70–74 y (14), 75–79 y (10)	2.4 m from the subject	**Concurrent (WBB)** CoM sway area $r = 0.93$ **Construct** (Johns Hopkins fall assessment scale) CoM sway area $\quad$ 65–69 y $\rho = 0.85$, $\quad$ 70–74 y $\rho = 0.89$, $\quad$ 75–79 y $\rho = 0.93$	—	M/N

Abbreviations: 1LST, single leg stance test; 2LST, double legs stance test; 3DMA, 3D motion analysis system; AP/ML, anteroposterior/mediolateral movement plane; CoM, center of body mass; displ, displacement; EC, eyes closed; EDSS, expanded disability status scale; EO, eyes open; flex, flexion; FRT, functional reach test; FTSTS, Five times sit to stand; HA, healthy adults (young and middle-aged); H/M/L, study of high/medium/low quality; lat, lateral; ICC, intraclass correlation coefficient; LBP, patients with low back pain; MA, master athletes; MS, patients with multiple sclerosis; MSWS-12, 12-item MS walking scale questionnaire; OA, older adults; SVmax, maximal sway velocity; SVx, mean sway velocity; r, Pearson correlation coefficient; YA, young adults; YBT, Y-balance test; Y/N, yes/no recommendation /available; ρ, Spearman correlation coefficient.

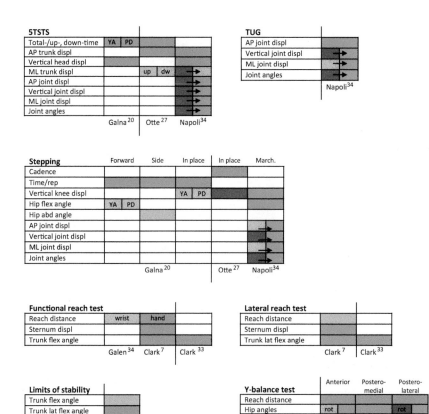

Fig. 2. Criterion validity of 5TSTS test, TUG test, stepping, and dynamic balance tests (functional reach tests, lateral reach test, limits of stability, Y-balance test) using the Kinect: vertical lines separate Kinect versions 1 and 2. Arrow represents range of validity values. abd, abduction; AP/ML, anteroposterior/mediolateral movement plane; displ, displacement; dw, down; flex, flexion; lat, lateral; PD, patients with Parkinson disease; rep, repetition; rot, rotations; YA, young adults.

The strengths of the criterion validity and the reliability of the transitional movements, stepping, and dynamic balance tests are summarized in **Figs. 2** and **3** respectively.

The strengths of the criterion validity and the reliability of the static balance tests are summarized in **Figs. 4** and **5** respectively.

Methodological quality of 9 studies[7–9,27–29,31,32,33] was rated as high, 10 studies[20,30,35–39,41–43] were medium, and 2[33,34,40] of low quality. Eight studies[7,9,27–31] were recommended for clinical use as an outcome measure. Software was not available for clinical use, but 4 groups of investigators would share it for research.[8,20,27,31,35,42,43]

DISCUSSION

The purpose of this article is to evaluate the validity and reliability of using the Kinect camera as an assessment tool for transitional movement and balance. Further, the authors sought to recommend the use of the Kinect as a tool for practice. To recommend

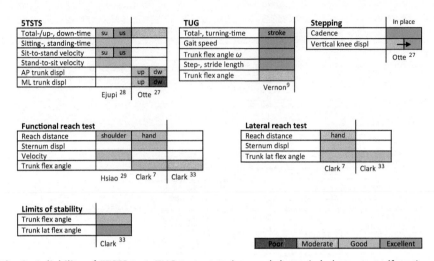

Fig. 3. Reliability of 5TSTS test, TUG test, stepping, and dynamic balance tests (functional reach tests, lateral reach test, limits of stability, Y-balance test) using the Kinect: vertical lines separate Kinect versions 1 and 2. Arrow represents range of reliability values. Stroke, patients after stroke; su, supervised; us, unsupervised.

the tool for practice, the study needed to report both validity and reliability. The authors accepted criterion validity tested against a gold standard 3DMA or a force plate or concurrent validity tested relative to the standardized clinical test. Many more studies reported validity alone than reliability, which limited the application to practice. In addition, studies that had both validity and reliability of high strength were further investigated for their realistic application to practice by contacting the investigators about their willingness to share their software. We discuss the findings, make specific recommendations for practice, and then comment on the challenges with this type of research and the translation into practice.

Transitional Movements, Stepping, and Dynamic Balance Tests

Criterion validity of Kinect temporal and spatial parameters for transitional movements, stepping,[20,27,34] and dynamic balance tests[7,33,37] was generally excellent or good. However, there were some exceptions for forward reach distance,[35] displacements in mediolateral (ML)[27,34] or vertical movement planes,[20,27,34] and joint angles.[20,34,37] These results are similar to those reported for the criterion validity of Kinect for temporal and displacement gait parameters.[19] Kinematics measured in the sagittal plane, reported in these studies, are more robust than those in other planes. The reported reliability of Kinect temporal and spatial parameters for transitional movements,[9,28] stepping,[27] and dynamic balance tests[7,29,33] were also generally good to excellent. There were some exceptions for temporal,[27] spatial (trunk and hand displacements),[7,27] and kinematic (trunk angles) parameters.[33] The V2 Kinect camera was successful in discriminating with center of body mass (CoM) displacement between young and older adults,[42,43] and the mean velocity of sit to stand was the best discriminator when using the V1 camera between the fallers and nonfallers based on 12-month retrospective fall data.[28] Discriminant validity between low-risk and high-risk fallers was supported for temporal and spatial parameters of the TUG.[39]

Recommendations for practice using these tests as an outcome measure:

- Using the V1 camera for:
  - Total time and sit-to-stand velocity for the 5TSTS[28]
  - Total time to perform the TUG[9]
  - All parameters of the functional reach test (FRT)[7,29]
  - Sternum displacement and lateral trunk flexion angle for the lateral reach test[7]
- Using the V2 camera for:
  - Up and down time, and anteroposterior (AP) trunk displacement[27] for the 5TSTS
  - Cadence during stepping in place[27]
  - Lateral trunk flexion angle for the lateral reach test
  - Trunk flexion and trunk lateral flexion angle during limits of stability

Using the recommended tests in practice may not be possible. Clark and colleagues,[33] and (Clark RA, personal communication, 2018) whose work was recommended for the TUG, FRT,[7] and limits of stability using both the V1 and V2 camera, was interested in principle in sharing the software; however, he thought it was not efficient supplying and updating the code because Microsoft has discontinued the production of the camera (Clark RA, personal communication, 2018). Otte and colleagues'[27] work is part of a company called Motognosis. They were willing to share their software for research and may have a commercial product in 2019. Of the recommended tests, we were unable to contact Ejupi and colleagues[28] and Hsiao and colleagues.[29] Further, investigators such as Leightley and colleagues,[42,43] whose tests were not recommend for practice because they did not report reliability, nevertheless

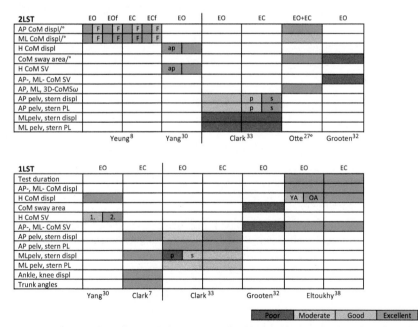

Fig. 4. Criterion validity of static balance tests; double-leg stance test (2LST) and single-leg stance test (1LST) using the Kinect: vertical lines separate Kinect versions 1 and 2. ap, feet apart; CoM, center of body mass; EC, eyes closed; EO, eyes open; f, foam; F, force plate; H, horizontal movement plane; OA, older adults; pelv/p, pelvis; PL, path length; stern/s, sternum; SV, sway velocity; Sω, sway angular velocity.

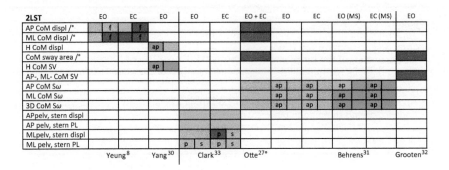

Fig. 5. Reliability of static balance tests; 2LST, tandem stance test (ST), and 1LST using the Kinect: vertical lines separate Kinect versions 1 and 2. HA, healthy adults; MS, patients with multiple sclerosis.

showed validity that was high and they were willing to share their software, whereas Dubois and colleagues[39] did not respond to our emails.

Static Balance Tests

Comparison between studies was challenging because there was a high degree of variability in the reporting of temporal and spatial parameters. Importantly, criterion validity of the Kinect for static balance assessment was good or excellent for all the parameters.[7,8,27,30,36,38] Validity of the pelvic and sternal parameters was good to excellent in anteroposterior (AP) directions, but lower in ML directions.[33] The results for velocity were mixed, with strong validity for linear velocity of CoM sway in horizontal[30] but not in AP and ML directions.[32] Concurrent validity was similar for both single-limb and double-limb stance conditions.[30,32,33]

Results for within-session or test-retest reliability testing were mixed both for spatial and temporal parameters and type of camera of static balance tests. Further, there is not a lot of redundancy for testing across studies. Good to excellent within-session reliability for horizontal CoM displacement and linear velocity of CoM sway of double-leg and single-leg stance tests were reported in a single study.[30] However, AP and ML CoM displacements and sway area,[8,27] and AP and ML pelvis and sternum displacements,[33] were generally unreliable, as were the CoM sway in AP and ML directions.[32] Reliability of 3D CoM sway angular velocity during double-leg and tandem stance test was generally good, and better than in AP and ML directions.[27,31] Reliability for double-leg stance test was generally better than tandem stance test.[31] However, comparison between double-leg and single-leg stance tests showed no clear pattern of reliability,[33] or it was poor in both conditions.[32] There was no clear difference in the reported reliability of the two Kinect versions. Reliability may have been influenced by the length of the time used to collect the data. For stabilometry, it is recommended that acquisition intervals be no less than 25 seconds,[44] and even as long as 90 seconds for double-leg stance.[45] In the studies in this review the intervals varied from 3 to 5[32] up to 60 seconds.[8] Single-leg stance was commonly captured for 15 seconds.[7,30,33] In 2 studies, data capturing combined both visual conditions in 1 interval,[27,31] and thus reached a minimum of time required. In 2 studies in this review,[32,33] a low acquisition time may also have influenced the validity. Similar findings of low validity were reported for WBB when double-leg test duration was less than 30 seconds.[2]

Testing static balance under different conditions, such as eyes open or closed, or manipulating the support surface had only a small influence on the validity of the tests. A small improvement in validity was observed in the eyes closed compared with the eyes open conditions.[8,33,38] Criterion validity was reported to be good to excellent for double-leg stance when tested standing on foam.[8] The excellent criterion validity was measured relative to the 3DMA, which was superior to the good criterion validity measured with a force plate (center of pressure).[8] This result must be viewed with caution as only 1 study in this review measured balance conditions on foam, which is in contrast with a review[2] of using foam on the WBB that included multiple studies in which the results were variable. In addition, studies that used the Kinect V1 showed consistent good to excellent validity for static balance compared with only a few studies with the V2 camera. Manipulation of vision had mixed results on the reliability of the measurements, whereas the use of foam decreased it. From the studies that compared eyes open and eyes closed test conditions,[8,31,33] there was no clear influence on reliability in either visual condition. These findings are similar to those reported for the WBB.[2] Reliability of the Kinect was generally poor for standing on the foam and lower than for a firm surface.[8] Similarly a trend of lower reliability for standing on a compliant rather than a firm surface was reported for stabilometry.[45]

Discriminant validity was assessed to distinguish between healthy adults and individuals with MS,[31] low back pain,[32] and different ages and abilities.[43] As expected, all 3 CoM sway velocities during eyes open and eyes closed conditions of double-leg stance test and tandem test were significantly higher for patients with MS than healthy adults. This difference was most pronounced in the feet together with eyes closed condition.[31] Similarly, AP and ML CoM displacements were significantly higher in older adults than in young adults and master athletes for the double-leg stance test, semitandem, and tandem stance tests, performed with eyes open.[43] For persons with low back pain, AP CoM sway velocity with eyes open was significantly higher than for healthy adults.[32] Manipulation of vision during single-leg stance further reinforced the pattern that ML and AP CoM displacements of young adults were significantly lower than those of older adults. With eyes closed, single-limb stance differentiated between the master athletes and the young adults.[43] These findings verified the Kinect measurements' ability to discriminate groups based on health condition and the complexity of the tested task.

Recommendations for practice using them as outcome measures:

- Using the V1 camera to measure:
  - Single-limb stance horizontal CoM displacement and sway velocity with eyes open[30]
  - Double-limb stance horizontal CoM displacement and sway velocity with eyes open[30]
- Using the V2 camera for:
  - Double-limb stance AP pelvis and sternum displacement and path length with eyes open and closed
  - Double-limb stance for ML and 3D CoM sway angular velocity with eyes open and closed with healthy adults and persons who have MS[27,31]

Access to the tests

As noted earlier Clark and colleagues[33] and (Clark RA, personal communication, 2018) thought that sharing the code was not worthwhile given the discontinuation of production of the Kinect V1.[7,9,33] Otte and colleagues'[27] and Behrens and colleagues'[31] work using Motognosis may result in a commercial product. Yeung and colleagues[8] are willing to share their software for research.

Note that reliability of the 3DMA systems varied relative to the Kinect. Five studies in this review also assessed the within-session[7,8,27,30] or test-retest[33] reliability of the criterion reference 3DMA. In general, it showed similar values to Kinect V1 or V2 for 5TSTS, stepping,[27] FRT[7] lateral reach test,[7,33] double-leg stance test,[8,27,30] and single-leg[7,30] stance tests. However, reliability of the 3DMA system was higher than that of Kinect for vertical knee displacement during stepping[27]; trunk flexion angle during FRT[33]; lateral reach test distance[7]; and for ankle, knee,[7] sternal, and pelvic[33] displacements during single-leg stance test. The 3DMA system showed larger estimates of reliability values than Kinect for the double-leg stance test.[33] However, reliability of the 3DMA system was lower than that of Kinect for trunk lateral flexion angle during limits of stability,[33] and AP CoM displacement during double-leg stance test,[8] with V2 and V1 respectively. Also, reliability of the criterion reference force plate for AP center of pressure displacement during double-leg stance test was lower than reliability of CoM displacement measured with Kinect.[8] Similar findings were reported for reliability between force plates and WBB.[2]

Interactive visual feedback information was given to subjects during the execution of some of the tests.[28,32,35] Several investigators performed the standardized tests using interactive visual feedback. An avatar was used as feedback when people performed 5TSTS and a virtual distance was represented for the FRT. These representations augment the standardized test, although the test may no longer be valid because the original procedures were not followed. However, it is not clear whether this augmented information improved the validity or reliability of the tests. The validation of interactive tests requires further study.

Limitations of the review

This article uses adapted COSMIN criteria.[22] The authors also created our own guidelines for what we determined was clinically acceptable. This guideline required that both validity and reliability be reported for a test and that they be of sufficient strength to recommend it. There is a chance that this stringent requirement may overlook a valuable study. However, we emailed investigators who had medium-quality studies in which reliability was not reported to query them about those tests. We were able to confirm in most cases that reliability was not tested. We also accepted a study with 9 subjects,[30] even though our criteria required 10 subjects. We made the decision that the quality of the study and the strength of the results were so strong that we would make an exception to the criteria. An additional limitation of the review is the inability to purely isolate the quality of the specific Kinect camera version because interpretation of the quality of the studies is confounded by the influence of the camera and the software used to analyze the data. We only searched 3 databases, which may have resulted in missing some studies. However, we selected both clinical (PubMed and CINAHL) and technical (IEEE) databases to reduce the likelihood of missing relevant studies.

Challenges with applications to practice

There are several challenges to applying the findings to practice. There is limited redundancy of the findings. There are also a limited number of recommended studies, those we rated as high quality, that reported good or excellent validity and reliability. To translate those findings into practice, the algorithms that were developed by the researchers to analyze the camera results would need to be shared. We found that a few investigators were willing to share their software for research,[8,27] and others thought that their software was outdated and could not support updating it because of competing time commitments,[42,43] plans to continue to update the software,[35] plans to commercialize the software,[27,31] or the decision that it was not worth the effort given that the camera will be discontinued.[7,33] We speculate that sharing the software would not be enough to translate the findings into practice. Likely, there will need to be a user interface that is accessible and easy to use as well as some training of clinicians who may want to adopt this technology into practice. This work is standard practice in the development of user interfaces that will be useful to health professionals and easy to understand by patients.[46–49] An additional barrier to translating these findings into practice is the existence of 2 versions of the Kinect camera. The results of this systematic review cannot definitively recommend the V1 or the V2 camera, further complicating a clinic's decision to purchase such a camera. The final challenge is knowing where to find the software if it is to be shared. The Open Rehabilitation Initiative (https://neurorehabilitation.m-iti.org/openrehab/) is an online community that seeks to share simulation that has been validated and shown to be reliable for both assessment and intervention.[50] It currently houses a single posturography simulation using the WBB.[51]

Considerations for Future Research

Based on this systematic review with a focus not just on validating off-the-shelf sensing devices for standardized assessments of motor performance but also applying them to practice, the authors strongly recommend that investigators report both validity and reliability. Further, if the field is to move forward with efficient research, it may be wise to find consistent ways of sharing software, whether it be for research or practice. Several investigators have shared their software either on their personal pages or GitHub.[42,43] A standard way of reporting our willingness to share software whether for research or eventually practice may be needed in these types of articles. If the Open Rehabilitation Initiative were to gain traction and be a credible resource for sharing knowledge and simulations, it may accelerate research and ultimately transfer the findings into practice.

SUMMARY

Criterion validity and reliability have been reported for standardized assessments such as the 5TSTS, the TUG, the FRT, and static balance tests. The results support the use of both the Kinect V1 and V2 cameras for selected temporal, spatial, and kinematic measures. However, there are limitation in the measurements. Translation into practice is limited by access to the software to run the tests.

REFERENCES

1. Breedon P, Siena L. Enhancing the measurement of clinical outcomes using Microsoft Kinect. IEEE Trans Neural Syst Rehabil Eng 2016;61–9. https://doi.org/10.1109/iTAG.2016.17.
2. Clark RA, Mentiplay BF, Pua YH, et al. Reliability and validity of the Wii Balance Board for assessment of standing balance: a systematic review. Gait Posture 2018;61:40–54.
3. Ruff J, Wang TL, Quatman-Yates CC, et al. Commercially available gaming systems as clinical assessment tools to improve value in the orthopaedic setting: a systematic review. Injury 2015;46(2):178–83.
4. Morrison C, Culmer P, Mentis H, et al. Vision-based body tracking: turning Kinect into a clinical tool. Disabil Rehabil Assist Technol 2016;11(6):516–20.
5. Mousavi Hondori H, Khademi M. A review on technical and clinical impact of Microsoft Kinect on physical therapy and rehabilitation. J Med Eng 2014;2014:846514.
6. Knippenberg E, Verbrugghe J, Lamers I, et al. Markerless motion capture systems as training device in neurological rehabilitation: a systematic review of their use, application, target population and efficacy. J Neuroeng Rehabil 2017;14(1):61.
7. Clark RA, Pua YH, Fortin K, et al. Validity of the Microsoft Kinect for assessment of postural control. Gait Posture 2012;36(3):372–7.
8. Yeung LF, Cheng KC, Fong CH, et al. Evaluation of the Microsoft Kinect as a clinical assessment tool of body sway. Gait Posture 2014;40(4):532–8.
9. Vernon S, Paterson K, Bower K, et al. Quantifying individual components of the timed up and go using the Kinect in people living with stroke. Neurorehabil Neural Repair 2015;29(1):48–53.
10. Nathan D, Huynh du Q, Rubenson J, et al. Estimating physical activity energy expenditure with the Kinect Sensor in an exergaming environment. PLoS One 2015;10(5):e0127113.
11. Mentiplay BF, Hasanki K, Perraton LG, et al. Three-dimensional assessment of squats and drop jumps using the Microsoft Xbox One Kinect: reliability and validity. J Sports Sci 2018;36(19):2202–9.
12. Kim WS, Cho S, Baek D, et al. Upper extremity functional evaluation by Fugl-Meyer assessment scoring using depth-sensing camera in hemiplegic stroke patients. PLoS One 2016;11(7):e0158640.
13. Simonsen D, Nielsen IF, Spaich EG, et al. Design and test of an automated version of the modified Jebsen test of hand function using Microsoft Kinect. J Neuroeng Rehabil 2017;14(1):38.
14. Lee S, Lee YS, Kim J. Automated evaluation of upper-limb motor function impairment using Fugl-Meyer assessment. IEEE Trans Neural Syst Rehabil Eng 2018;26(1):125–34.
15. Ma AJ, Rawat N, Reiter A, et al. Measuring patient mobility in the ICU using a novel noninvasive sensor. Crit Care Med 2017;45(4):630–6.
16. Yang MT, Chuang MW. Fall risk assessment and early-warning for toddler behaviors at home. Sensors (Basel) 2013;13(12):16985–7005.

17. Stone E, Skubic M, Rantz M, et al. Average in-home gait speed: investigation of a new metric for mobility and fall risk assessment of elders. Gait Posture 2015; 41(1):57–62.
18. Plantard P, Shum HPH, Le Pierres AS, et al. Validation of an ergonomic assessment method using Kinect data in real workplace conditions. Appl Ergon 2017; 65:562–9.
19. Springer S, Yogev Seligmann G. Validity of the Kinect for gait assessment: a focused review. Sensors (Basel) 2016;16(2):194.
20. Galna B, Barry G, Jackson D, et al. Accuracy of the Microsoft Kinect sensor for measuring movement in people with Parkinson's disease. Gait Posture 2014; 39(4):1062–8.
21. Geerse DJ, Coolen BH, Roerdink M. Kinematic validation of a multi-Kinect v2 instrumented 10-meter walkway for quantitative gait assessments. PLoS One 2015; 10(10):e0139913.
22. Terwee CB, Mokkink LB, Knol DL, et al. Rating the methodological quality in systematic reviews of studies on measurement properties: a scoring system for the COSMIN checklist. Qual Life Res 2012;21(4):651–7.
23. Portney LG, Watkins MP. Foundations of clinical research: applications to practice. Upper Saddle River (NJ): Pearson/Prentice Hall; 2009.
24. Koo TK, Li MY. A guideline of selecting and reporting intraclass correlation coefficients for reliability research. J Chiropr Med 2016;15(2):155–63.
25. Funaya H, Shibata T, Wada Y, et al. Accuracy assessment of Kinect body tracker in instant posturography for balance disorders. presented at the 7th International Symposium on Medical Information and Communication Technology (ISMICT). IEEE 2013;213–7.
26. Hotrabhavanananda B, Mishra AK, Skubic M, et al. Evaluation of the Microsoft Kinect skeletal versus depth data analysis for the timed up and go and figure 8 walk tests. Conf Proc IEEE Eng Med Biol Soc 2016;2016:2274–7.
27. Otte K, Kayser B, Mansow-Model S, et al. Accuracy and reliability of the Kinect version 2 for clinical measurement of motor function. PLoS One 2016;11(11): e0166532.
28. Ejupi A, Gschwind YJ, Brodie M, et al. Kinect-based choice reaching and stepping reaction time tests for clinical and in-home assessment of fall risk in older people: a prospective study. Eur Rev Aging Phys Act 2016;13:2.
29. Hsiao MY, Li CM, Lu IS, et al. An investigation of the use of the Kinect system as a measure of dynamic balance and forward reach in the elderly. Clin Rehabil 2018; 32(4):473–82.
30. Yang Y, Pu F, Li Y, et al. Reliability and validity of kinect RGB-D sensor for assessing standing balance. IEEE Sensors 2014;14(5):1633–8.
31. Behrens JR, Mertens S, Kruger T, et al. Validity of visual perceptive computing for static posturography in patients with multiple sclerosis. Mult Scler 2016;22(12): 1596–606.
32. Grooten WJA, Sandberg L, Ressman J, et al. Reliability and validity of a novel Kinect-based software program for measuring posture, balance and side-bending. BMC Musculoskelet Disord 2018;19(1):6.
33. Clark RA, Pua YH, Oliveira CC, et al. Reliability and concurrent validity of the Microsoft Xbox One Kinect for assessment of standing balance and postural control. Gait Posture 2015;42(2):210–3.
34. Napoli A, Glass S, Ward C, et al. Performance analysis of a generalized motion capture system using Microsoft Kinect 2.0. Biomed Signal Process Control 2017;38:265–80.

35. Galen SS, Pardo V, Wyatt D, et al. Validity of an interactive functional reach test. Games Health J 2015;4(4):278–84.
36. Chakravarty K, Suman S, Bhowmick B, et al. Quantification of balance in single limb stance using kinect. Presented at the IEEE International Conference on Acoustics, Speech and Signal Processing (ICASSP). IEEE 2016;854–8.
37. Eltoukhy M, Kuenze C, Oh J, et al. Kinect-based assessment of lower limb kinematics and dynamic postural control during the star excursion balance test. Gait Posture 2017;58:421–7.
38. Eltoukhy MA, Kuenze C, Oh J, et al. Validation of static and dynamic balance assessment using Microsoft Kinect for young and elderly populations. IEEE J Biomed Health Inform 2018;22(1):147–53.
39. Dubois A, Bihl T, Bresciani J-P. Automating the timed up and go test using a depth camera. Sensors (Basel) 2017;18(1):14.
40. Choi JS, Kang DW, Seo JW, et al. The development and evaluation of a program for leg-strengthening exercises and balance assessment using Kinect. J Phys Ther Sci 2016;28(1):33–7.
41. Mazumder O, Tripathy S, Roy S, et al. Postural sway based geriatric fall risk assessment using Kinect. IEEE Sensors 2017;1–3. https://doi.org/10.1109/ICSENS.2017.8234214.
42. Leightley D, Yap MH. Digital analysis of sit-to-stand in masters athletes, healthy old people, and young adults using a depth sensor. Healthcare (Basel) 2018;6(1) [pii:E21].
43. Leightley D, Yap MH, Coulson J, et al. Postural stability during standing balance and sit-to-stand in master athlete runners compared with nonathletic old and young adults. J Aging Phys Act 2017;25(3):345–50.
44. Scoppa F, Capra R, Gallamini M, et al. Clinical stabilometry standardization: basic definitions – acquisition interval – sampling frequency. Gait Posture 2010;37:290–2.
45. Ruhe A, Fejer R, Walker B. The test-retest reliability of centre of pressure measures in bipedal static task conditions–a systematic review of the literature. Gait Posture 2010;32(4):436–45.
46. Proffitt R, Lange B. Considerations in the efficacy and effectiveness of virtual reality interventions for stroke rehabilitation: moving the field forward. Phys Ther 2015;95(3):441–8.
47. Deutsch JE, Lewis JA, Burdea G. Technical and patient performance using a virtual reality-integrated telerehabilitation system: preliminary finding. IEEE Trans Neural Syst Rehabil Eng 2007;15(1):30–5.
48. Lewis JA, Deutsch JE, Burdea G. Usability of the remote console for virtual reality telerehabilitation: formative evaluation. Cyberpsychol Behav 2006;9(2):142–7.
49. Morrison C, D'Souza M, Huckvale K, et al. Usability and acceptability of ASSESS MS: assessment of motor dysfunction in multiple sclerosis using depth-sensing computer vision. JMIR Hum Factors 2015;2(1):e11.
50. Bermudez i Badia S, Deutsch JE, Llorens R. Open rehabilitation initiative: design and formative evaluation. In: Sharkey P, Rizzo AA, editors. Proceedings of the 11th international conference on disability, virtual reality and associated technologies (ICDVRAT 2016). Reading (UK): University of Reading; 2016. p. 93–100.
51. Llorens R, Latorre J, Noe E, et al. Posturography using the Wii Balance Board: a feasibility study with healthy adults and adults post-stroke. Gait Posture 2016;43:228–32.

Advances in Prosthetics and Rehabilitation of Individuals with Limb Loss

Mary S. Keszler, MD[a,b], Jeffrey T. Heckman, DO[a,b],
G. Eli Kaufman, CPO[a,c], David C. Morgenroth, MD[a,b,c],*

KEYWORDS

• Prosthetics • Amputation • Rehabilitation • Limb loss • Function

KEY POINTS

• Surgical decision-making and postamputation rehabilitation are important and often overlooked elements of postamputation function and quality of life.
• Advances in prosthetic componentry often aim to replicate functional aspects of the biologic limb.
• The postamputation course and a prosthesis prescription is unique to each individual and the individual's needs, goals, and abilities.

INTRODUCTION

Approximately 1.6 million people in the United States are currently living with limb loss, a population projected to more than double by 2050.[1] Amputation results in a wide range of functional limitations; advances in surgical, rehabilitative, and prosthetic care are aimed at optimizing functional quality of life for the spectrum of individuals with limb loss.

Disclosure Statement: M.S. Keszler's contributions were supported by the Office of Academic Affiliations, Department of Veterans Affairs. J.T. Heckman's contributions were supported by the VHA Amputation System of Care. D.C. Morgenroth's contributions were supported by the VA Puget Sound Health Care System, Seattle, WA. G.E. Kaufman's contributions were supported by the VA RR&D Center for Limb Loss and Mobility. This material is the result of work supported with resources and the use of facilities at the VA Puget Sound Health Care System. The contents of this article do not represent the views of the US Department of Veterans Affairs or the US government.

[a] Division of Rehabilitation Care Services, VA Puget Sound Health Care System, 1660 South Columbian Way, S-117-RCS, Seattle, WA 98108, USA; [b] Department of Rehabilitation Medicine, University of Washington, Seattle, WA, USA; [c] Center for Limb Loss and Mobility (CLiMB), Department of Veterans Affairs, Office of Research and Development, Seattle, WA, USA
* Corresponding author. VA Puget Sound Health Care Service, S-117-RCS, 1660 South Columbian Way, Seattle, WA 98108.
E-mail address: dmorgen@uw.edu

Phys Med Rehabil Clin N Am 30 (2019) 423–437
https://doi.org/10.1016/j.pmr.2018.12.013
1047-9651/19/Published by Elsevier Inc.

Prosthetic limbs are often an important element to functional restoration. The use of prosthetics dates back at least 3500 years to ancient Egypt, but prosthetic technology remained relatively stagnant until the nineteenth century. Significant advancement in the field of prosthetics has greatly accelerated during the past few decades. Although these technological advancements tend to capture the imagination and media attention, optimal surgical and rehabilitative care play an equally vital yet often underappreciated role in enabling functional restoration after amputation.

We therefore structured this narrative review to initially concentrate on advances in surgical and rehabilitative care. This is followed by noteworthy advances in prosthetics, including potential advantages and disadvantages of each. Our goal is to herein provide an overview of important recent advances in the field of amputation rehabilitation and prosthetics (attempting to minimize focal overlap with prior narrative reviews[2–4]), citing evidence where available, and providing clinicians with information that they may consider using in clinical practice.

SURGICAL ADVANCES

The choice of amputation level and the quality of amputation surgery strongly influence subsequent functional restoration and prosthetic fitting. Amputation level determination ideally includes surgical, physiatric, and prosthetic input, weighing factors such as healing potential, re-amputation risk, and functional implications at each amputation level being considered.

The AMPREDICT tool was developed by Czerniecki and colleagues[5] to aid in predicting mobility, morbidity, and mortality, as a means of weighing the likely risks and benefits at a given level of amputation during preoperative planning. They reported that older age, history of chronic obstructive pulmonary disease, diabetes mellitus, depression or anxiety, and poor to fair self-rated health reduce the chance of achieving basic mobility.[5] Qualities that lead to an increased likelihood of achieving basic mobility and independence with advanced mobility include more distal amputation (for predicting basic mobility), increased body mass index up to 30 kg/m^2, being white, married, and having a high school education.[5]

Predicting the most appropriate amputation level remains challenging, especially in medically complex patients with dysvascular disease. A relatively common scenario in this patient population is deciding whether to perform a partial foot amputation (PFA) or a transtibial amputation (TTA). A recent systematic review revealed 42% of individuals suffered perioperative complications following PFA, including wound dehiscence or necrosis and reamputation, compared with 28% of those with TTA.[6] Quality of life and mobility were similar between the 2 groups, and although those with TTA had higher mortality rates, it is unknown if this was a consequence of amputation level or more advanced disease states.[6] Shared decision-making resources are being developed to help providers weigh probable outcomes with patients' priorities when it comes to determining amputation level.[7]

In addition to advances in amputation level decision making, novel surgical techniques have been developed with the goal of improving function and quality of life in subgroups of this patient population. For example, upper limb composite allotransplantation aims to provide sensation, proprioception, and intuitive control. As of 2015, the survival rate of 103 individuals who underwent isolated upper limb transplantation was 98.5% and overall graft survival was 88.3%, with poor outcomes in 4 individuals who underwent combined transplants.[8] Although these results are promising, successfully maintaining a transplanted limb requires strict compliance with lifelong immunosuppression and participation in arduous courses of physical and occupational therapy. To improve compliance with immunosuppression, a simplified regimen has been developed; of 5 patients studied, those on this new regimen experienced infrequent and reversible skin rejections and minor wound infections.[9] Regarding upper extremity (UE) function, individuals who made significant improvements tended to be patients with greater intrinsic muscle function and those with more distal amputations of their nondominant hand.[10,11] One must consider a multitude of factors (eg, residual limb length and health, other comorbidities or injuries, hand dominance) when considering allotransplantation. Consequently, this surgical option is currently appropriate for only a very select group of individuals.

Targeted muscle reinnervation (TMR) is a surgical technique intended to enable more intuitive control of UE myoelectric prostheses and to potentially reduce pain (eg, neuroma), by coopting residual nerves to muscles that have lost function.[12] Kuiken and colleagues,[13] who developed this technique, had a 95% nerve transfer success rate with 25 of 27 patients successfully fit with TMR-controlled devices. After this procedure, approximately 79% of those with phantom limb pain had an exacerbation that generally abated in 4 to 6 weeks and approximately 86% of those with symptomatic neuromas became symptom-free.[13] Functionally, these patients showed improvement on multiple tests of UE function compared with preoperative function with a conventional myoelectric prosthesis.[13] Although TMR carries relatively low risk and has clear potential benefits, candidacy for TMR must be carefully considered; potential candidates must be without concomitant nerve injuries and willing to undergo rigorous training. Expectations also must be managed, as many individuals having undergone TMR surgery continue to demonstrate superior functional outcomes using body-powered devices.

Osseointegration is a procedure in which an implant is secured within the shaft of the long bone of the residual limb. An abutting percutaneous fixture allows for assembly of modular prosthetic components, thereby eliminating the need for a socket. Osseointegration may enable prosthesis use for individuals who are not able to achieve a sufficiently comfortable socket fit. In addition, due to the absence of a soft tissue–socket interface, osseointegration may provide improved proprioception and reduced energy expenditure when compared with conventional prostheses. However, the potential for complications must be considered; in a study involving individuals with transhumeral amputations, the implant survival rate was 80% at 5 years and the most common adverse event was superficial infection of the skin penetration site with an incidence of 38% at 5 years.[14] In a study involving subjects with transfemoral amputations, approximately 18% were diagnosed with implant-associated osteomyelitis with a 10-year cumulative risk of 20%.[15] Approximately 11% required extraction of the implant with a 9% 10-year cumulative risk.[15] A recent systematic review found low-quality evidence of improvement in condition-specific quality of life, health, pain, wearing time, mobility, use of walking aids, energy costs of ambulation, hip range of motion (ROM), sitting comfort, and functional outcome measures in transfemoral amputees.[16] Another recent systematic review found improvements in pain and quality of life based on moderate-quality studies.[17] Clearly, osseointegration has the potential for substantial benefits in a select group of individuals (eg, compliant with treatment, healthy with good-quality bone at the residual limb, and without immunocompromising conditions); however, the potential benefits must be weighed against the significant potential for adverse events, such as implant failure and infection.

REHABILITATION ADVANCES

Physiatric-led, team-based rehabilitation is often an important element in optimizing functional outcomes and quality of life, with or without a prosthesis, in those with limb loss. In addition to restoring physical function, rehabilitation also should focus on the prevalent psychosocial sequelae of amputation. Because postamputation depression rates range from 18.0% to 28.7% and postamputation anxiety is also common (18.5% in one study), addressing mental health and emotional sequelae are important, although often overlooked, features of enhancing functional recovery.[18,19] Social integration, peer support, and visitation play a significant role in minimizing depressive symptoms and improving adjustment to disability. The combination of perceived lower levels of social support and increased requirement for assistance with activities of daily living at baseline is associated with depressive symptoms at 1 year.[20] In a longitudinal study examining postamputation social integration, a higher Multidimensional Scale of Perceived Social Support score at 1 month was associated with lower levels of pain interference, greater mobility, and greater levels of satisfaction with life at 1 month, as well as greater mobility and occupational function at 6 months.[21] Support from a caregiver also was associated with higher levels of life satisfaction, whereas caregiver-specific conflict was associated with lower levels of life satisfaction and higher levels of depression.[22]

For individuals who have experienced limb loss, other psychological constructs affected by depression and anxiety include pain and body image. The Trinity Amputation and Prosthesis Experience Scales (TAPES) is a self-report outcome measure used to assess psychosocial adjustment, activity restriction, and prosthesis satisfaction. Research using TAPES found that individuals who experienced residual limb or phantom limb pain were significantly less satisfied with the prosthesis and had difficulty adjusting to their disability compared with those without pain, but there was no difference in activity restriction.[23] Furthermore, anxiety and depression significantly correlate with body-image disturbance, as well as psychosocial and social adjustment and adjustment to disability on the TAPES.[18] These modifiable and nonmodifiable predictors for this specific patient population are important to understand so that early signs and symptoms can be noted and treated early, thereby improving mental health and long-term function.

An understanding of the benefits of exercise and sports for persons with disabilities, along with advances in wheelchair and prosthesis technology, have ushered in a vibrant culture for adaptive sports and has proven to be an important pathway to enhance physical and mental health in those with amputations. Individuals with traumatic lower limb loss demonstrated lower baseline maximal oxygen consumption, anaerobic threshold, and maximum workload compared with nonexercising controls, but demonstrated improvement with subsequent endurance training program.[24] Those involved in sports report enhanced quality of life, life satisfaction, and self-esteem.[25,26] Furthermore, those who exercise regularly report significantly better body-image compared with those who do not.[27] Adaptive sports for persons with limb loss has become readily available via local community organizations as well as national organizations, such as the US Department of Veterans Affairs and Challenged Athletes Foundation, as well as sports-specific clubs. Depending on a patient's specific interest, function, and general health, adaptive sports should be considered as part of a comprehensive rehabilitation program.

PROSTHESIS ADVANCES
Socket

A well-fitting socket is often considered the most critical component of a prosthesis; potential functional benefits of advanced prosthetic components will typically be lost when socket fit is suboptimal. High-quality socket design includes careful consideration of the residual limb (eg, skin properties, bony protuberances, nerve locations, underlying soft tissue quality), as well as the forces predicted to occur between the prosthesis and residual limb during a range of static and dynamic functional activities. Although skilled prosthetists are often able to achieve a comfortable socket fit even for patients with suboptimal residual limb properties, the trade-off is the inherent inconsistency in the custom socket design process.

Innovative attempts to standardize socket design while improving comfort and function include the High-Fidelity Interface System (HiFi; BioDesigns, Inc, Westlake Village, CA) and Marlo Anatomic Socket (MAS), each of which stipulate highly specified casting and modeling instructions. The HiFi design incorporates 4 longitudinal struts intended to maximize stability along the long bone(s) of the residual limb. The MAS, specifically for transfemoral prostheses, features a lowered anterior and posterior brim aimed at increasing hip ROM, potentially at the expense of residual limb-socket lever arm and stability.[28] The Northwestern University Flexible Subischial Vacuum (NU-FlexSIV) socket uses active vacuum suspension in an attempt to enhance reliability of suspension while maintaining the benefits of ROM and comfort.[29] NU-FlexSIV has demonstrated early success among a small cohort of patients with varying residual limb lengths.[29]

The fixed volume of traditional sockets can lead to challenges for prosthesis limb users who require accommodation for substantial volume fluctuations based on activity or comorbid medical conditions. Attempts to meet this challenge have led to the emergence of modular sockets. The RevoFit (WillowWood, Sterling, OH, and Click Medical, Steamboat Springs, CO) **(Fig. 1)**, adapted from the dial-string tightening system on modern ski boots, is an adjustable system that may be fabricated into an otherwise custom socket. By modulating the tension of a high-tensile string running through the socket walls, the wearer can tighten or loosen isolated areas of the socket as limb volume changes throughout the day. Further modularization is represented in socket designs by LIM Innovations (San Francisco, CA) and Martin Bionics (Oklahoma City, OK), both of which require minor custom fabrication **(Figs. 2 and 3)**. These modular sockets feature framelike structures with major segments that can be adjusted by the practitioner and fine-tuning adjustment components that allow the user to quickly adjust for daily residual limb volume changes.

Despite potential advances, there remain certain drawbacks to emerging socket technologies. The string used in the RevoFit, while generally strong, can fray and break

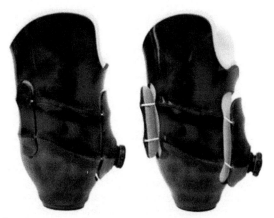

Fig. 1. RevoFit socket. (*Courtesy of* WillowWood, Sterling, OH.)

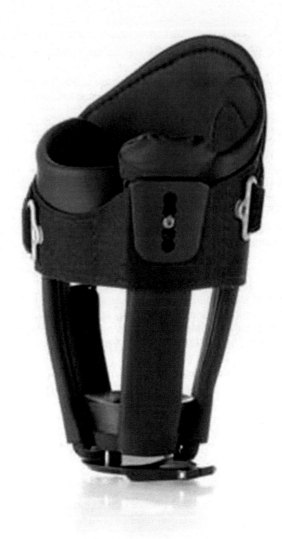

Fig. 2. Modular socket. (*Courtesy of* LIM Innovations, San Francisco, CA.)

during wear. It is recommended that the strings be evaluated and replaced every 6 months to avoid catastrophic failure. Successful modular socket use depends on the user accurately assessing when and how adjustments need to be made throughout the day. For this reason, modular sockets may not be suitable for individuals with cognitive, fine motor, or sensory impairment. Finally, modular solutions may work well in certain situations, but a custom socket design crafted by a skilled and experienced prosthetist remains the gold standard.

Fabrication

Several decades ago, the introduction of thermoplastics, composite materials, and endoskeletal components revolutionized the fabrication process, resulting in the near extinction of prosthetic limbs made from leather and carved wood. These materials and techniques, which have become industry standard, permit more rapid

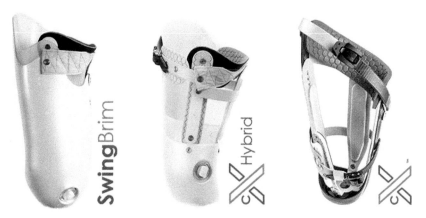

Fig. 3. Examples of different modular sockets. (*Courtesy of* Martin Bionics, Oklahoma City, OK.)

fabrication of prosthetic limbs with increased durability and adjustability, but carry certain constraints, including reliance on toxic materials, the requirement for skilled practitioners, and the need for considerable physical space to work and store plaster models.

Today, emerging digital technologies such as 3-dimensional (3D) scanning and printing offer the potential to address some of these issues, bringing enhanced safety, automation, and convenience to the fabrication process (**Figs. 4** and **5**). However, limitations of current digital scanning and 3D printing technology (eg, durability limitations, mapping the surface topography of the limb without capturing important underlying tissue characteristics) are important to consider. There are clearly trade-offs between traditional custom socket design and emerging technologies that increase automation and consistency.

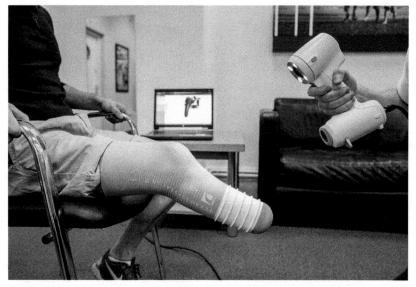

Fig. 4. 3D scanner. (*Courtesy of* Ability Matters, Avingdon, Oxfordshire, UK.)

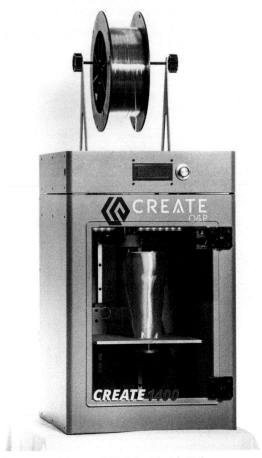

Fig. 5. 3D printer. (*Courtesy of* Create O&P, Lake Placid, NY.)

SUSPENSION AND INTERFACE

Safe and confident use of a prosthesis depends on reliable suspension. Some recent advancements have focused on simplifying donning techniques for individuals with visual and manual dexterity impairments. For example, the MagnoFlex (Ottobock, Duderstadt, Germany) magnetic and flexible pin suspension system is similar to a conventional pin-lock suspension system, but the pin is both magnetically attracted to the lock and articulated so that it does not need to be perfectly straight to engage (**Fig. 6**). Whereas a conventional pin-lock system requires good "aim" to engage the pin with the lock, the MagnoFlex system is much more forgiving. It might seem that this innovation should be universally beneficial; however, this system allows the prosthesis to be donned with increased imprecision. Although suspension may be secure, prosthesis orientation and fit may be compromised, and shear tension at the distal residual may be increased, particularly during high-activity conditions.

Common skin problems resulting from prostheses wear include contact dermatitis, epidermoid cysts, and bacterial or fungal infections.[30] Such problems are heavily impacted by the prosthesis interface (ie, the component of the device that directly contacts the skin). This is particularly true for lower extremity prostheses that require

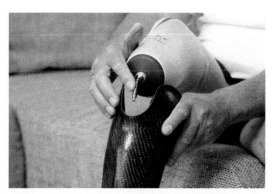

Fig. 6. Magnetic/flexible pin. (*Courtesy of* Ottobock, Duderstadt, Germany.)

that the wearer place full body weight through the socket. Due to their soft and flexible properties, gel liners can be effective at mitigating problems resulting from mechanical stresses on the skin; however, the insulative nature of gel liners can have adverse effects; heat buildup often triggers perspiration, and an accumulation of moisture can compromise liner adhesion and result in a sudden loss of suspension. To address this problem, manufacturers have developed gel liners containing many small perforations (**Fig. 7**). These full-thickness perforations allow moisture to move to the outside of the liner. Perforated gel liners may help to reduce moisture within the liner; however, the perforations in the liner walls can trap dirt and bacteria, creating an unhygienic environment and increased potential for a variety of skin problems. Perforated gel liners will likely work best for patients with perspiration-related problems who are fastidious in keeping their supplies clean.

LOWER EXTREMITY PROSTHETICS

Most advances in prosthetic feet have attempted to emulate functional properties of the biological foot-ankle system. Even with improvements in prosthetic foot design, there continue to be inevitable trade-offs such that no single foot is best for all individuals in all situations. An optimal prosthetic foot prescription matches mechanical and other properties of the prosthetic foot with an individual's goals, needs, and abilities, while minimizing trade-offs (eg, increased mobility often comes at the expense of decreased stability).

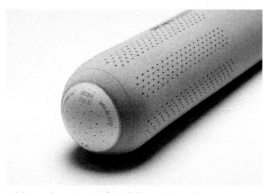

Fig. 7. Perforated gel liner. (*Courtesy of* Endolite, Miamisburg, OH.)

This balance in decision-making is exaggerated by sports-specific feet, such as those designed specifically for skiing or swimming. Although these can be indispensable to the avid athlete who needs to lock the foot directly into the ski or articulate the foot for wearing a fin, they are generally uncomfortable when used for other basic tasks, such as walking. The same can be said of running-specific feet, which store and return energy through bending of long C-shaped carbon fiber blades (**Fig. 8**); the higher level of stiffness required for running is uncomfortably rigid for walking, and the absence of a heel can impair balance. To address these shortcomings, crossover feet have emerged to enable walking and running with the same foot. Crossover feet feature a similarly long C-shaped blade, but with a heel component for improved standing stability and enabling a heel strike during walking (**Fig. 9**). When compared with a traditional energy-storing foot, a crossover foot was found to improve mobility, balance confidence, functional satisfaction, and lead to longer sound-side step lengths.[31] There was also a trend toward lower oxygen consumption at self-selected walking speeds[32]; however, in a small study there was no significant difference between crossover and energy-storing feet in low-level and high-level performance-based outcome measures.[33]

With advances in software and battery technology, microprocessor knees and feet can be beneficial for certain patients. Microprocessor knees typically provide variable resistance (many during both stance and swing phases), emulating eccentric muscular contractions. Some knees recognize deliberate user movements, initiating transitions

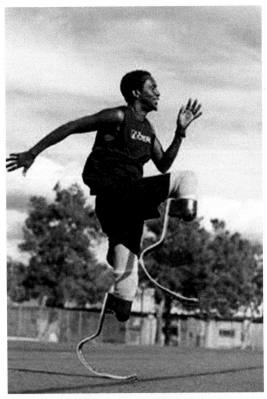

Fig. 8. Running foot. (*Courtesy of* Össur, Inc, Reykjavik, Iceland.)

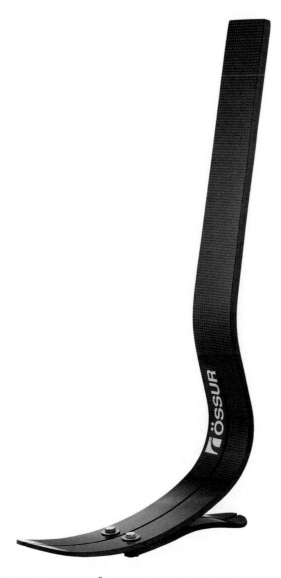

Fig. 9. Crossover foot. (*Courtesy of* Össur, Inc, Reykjavik, Iceland.)

to modified walking modes.[34] Specific modes, like stair mode, can be used not only as designed for ascending stairs with a symmetric step-over-step pattern, but also during activities, such as hiking when rapid preswing knee flexion is required to step over obstacles. In theory, advanced modes enhance mobility; however, approximately 30% of patients were unable to achieve safe utilization of stair mode despite advanced training.[34] Microprocessor-controlled powered feet can provide powered dorsiflexion during swing and push-off at the end of stance phase. Active dorsiflexion can help reduce fall risk by increasing toe clearance during walking and stair ascent, decrease energy cost of walking, and improve several functional outcomes in non-dysvascular individuals with TTA.[35,36] Powered push-off has been found to increase self-selected walking speed, reduce metabolic rate with level walking, increase power with step-to-step transition, and improve gait symmetry.[37–39] Risk of intact limb knee osteoarthritis may be reduced as well, as powered push-off can reduce contralateral knee loading.[40] Notable downsides of microprocessor and powered components include increased weight, cost, maintenance, and battery limitations.

UPPER EXTREMITY PROSTHETICS

Although as many as two-thirds of Americans with major UE amputations use body-powered prostheses, most recent advances have been made in externally powered devices.[1] Specific areas of development include prosthesis control strategies and expansion of independent joint mobility.

The first clinically significant myoelectric prosthesis was introduced in the 1960s, and until recently little had changed.[41] Traditional externally powered myoelectric prostheses require learned motor control strategies that are not necessarily intuitive (eg, activating wrist extensors opens the powered terminal device in a transradial amputee).

The recently introduced Coapt (Chicago, IL) pattern-recognition control system uses an array of up to 8 electrodes to perceive muscle activity patterns in the residuum. Rather than the wearer adapting to the system, the system learns which movements are intended based on user-specified patterns of muscle activation. Thus, control of a Coapt-equipped prosthesis is substantially more intuitive than a traditional myoelectric prosthesis. Coapt system calibration, which takes about a minute, must be performed as frequent as 1 to 2 times per day to maintain optimal performance. It is worth noting that control of traditional and pattern-recognition myoelectric systems can be enhanced by TMR surgery, as previously described.

Developers have also explored additional control strategies. For instance, the Mobius Bionics (Manchester, NH) Luke Arm can use an array of control mechanisms, including a wireless foot controller and End Point Control. The foot controller is an inertial measurement unit, which acts like a joystick controller for the prosthesis. End Point Control enables simultaneous coordinated movement in several joints to position the terminal device at a point in space (the end point) based on user commands.[42] Control strategies can be enhanced through feedback mechanisms, such as socket vibration.

Some commercially available externally powered prosthetic devices now also permit multiple degrees of freedom, or independent planar movement, at specific joints. This is particularly apparent in advanced terminal devices with 5 fully articulating digits capable of multiple grip patterns and conforming grasp. The shoulder-level Luke Arm features 10 powered motors and freedom of movement between the shoulder and forearm are comparable to the biological arm.

Despite these recent advances in powered prosthetics, significant limitations still exist. Although researchers are working on restoring sensory feedback, the current state of the art is far from accurately emulating this vital function of biological limbs; without sensory feedback, visual information becomes paramount, and is limited by typical myoelectric terminal devices. Control strategies may be more intuitive, but lag time between user input and device response remains. Each degree of freedom built into a prosthesis intended to improve function places a greater cognitive burden of training on the user. For these and other reasons (eg, increased weight and cost), many individuals still prefer body-powered prostheses and device abandonment rates remain high. The acceptance and optimal use of an upper-limb prosthesis is enhanced dramatically when a patient is involved with an upper-limb specialty program that incorporates expeditious prosthetic care and occupational therapy.[43]

SUMMARY

High-quality surgical and rehabilitative care are vital to optimize functional restoration, participation, and psychosocial well-being, while minimizing painful associated conditions and minimizing the likelihood of subsequent surgical revisions or contralateral amputations. An experienced, thoughtful, and communicative multidisciplinary team, often led by a physiatrist, is instrumental in maximizing functional quality of life throughout the life span for individuals with amputations.

Optimizing prosthetic prescription is thought to play an important role in maximizing function and satisfaction in prosthetic users; however, with the multitude of existing options to choose from, there is limited evidence to effectively guide the process.[44,45] In this review, we presented recent advances in prosthetics to help inform clinicians of ever-expanding available options. Because commercial prosthetic component designs and features have important functional trade-offs, the selection of an appropriate component is highly dependent on the unique needs, goals, and abilities of each individual patient. It is therefore important to stress that "more recent," "higher tech," or "more expensive" should not necessarily be equated with superior when it comes to prosthetic provision. Finally, optimizing surgical and rehabilitative care are vital components of enhancing functional recovery and quality of life in people with limb loss.

REFERENCES

1. Ziegler-Graham K, MacKenzie EJ, Ephraim PL, et al. Estimating the prevalence of limb loss in the United States: 2005 to 2050. Arch Phys Med Rehabil 2008;89(3): 422–9.
2. Esquenazi A. Amputation rehabilitation and prosthetic restoration. From surgery to community reintegration. Disabil Rehabil 2004;26(14–15):831–6.
3. Zlotolow DA, Kozin SH. Advances in upper extremity prosthetics. Hand Clin 2012; 28(4):587–93.
4. Kistenberg RS. Prosthetic choices for people with leg and arm amputations. Phys Med Rehabil Clin N Am 2014;25(1):93–115.
5. Czerniecki JM, Turner AP, Williams RM, et al. The development and validation of the AMPREDICT model for predicting mobility outcome after dysvascular lower extremity amputation. J Vasc Surg 2017;65(1):162–71.e3.
6. Dillon MP, Quigley M, Fatone S. Outcomes of dysvascular partial foot amputation and how these compare to transtibial amputation: a systematic review for the development of shared decision-making resources. Syst Rev 2017;6(54): 1–20.
7. Quigley M, Dillon MP, Fatone S. Development of shared decision-making resources to help inform difficult healthcare decisions: an example focused on dysvascular partial foot and transtibial amputations. Prosthet Orthot Int 2018. https:// doi.org/10.1177/0309364617752984.
8. Shores JT, Brandacher G, Lee WPA. Hand and upper extremity transplantation: an update of outcomes in the worldwide experience. Plast Reconstr Surg 2015; 135(2):351e–60e.
9. Schneeberger S, Gorantla VS, Brandacher G, et al. Upper-extremity transplantation using a cell-based protocol to minimize immunosuppression. Ann Surg 2014; 257(2):345–51.
10. Landin L, Bonastre J, Casado-Sanchez C, et al. Outcomes with respect to disabilities of the upper limb after hand allograft transplantation: a systematic review. Transpl Int 2012;25(4):424–32.

11. Pet MA, Morrison SD, Mack JS, et al. Comparison of patient-reported outcomes after traumatic upper extremity amputation: replantation versus prosthetic rehabilitation. Injury 2016;47(12):2783–8.

12. Cheesborough JE, Smith LH, Kuiken TA, et al. Targeted muscle reinnervation and advanced prosthetic arms. Semin Plast Surg 2015;29(1):62–72.

13. Kuiken TA, Feuser AES, Barlow AK, editors. Targeted muscle reinnveration: a neural interface for artificial limbs. Boca Raton (FL): CRC Press; 2014.

14. Tsikandylakis G, Berlin Ö, Brånemark R. Implant survival, adverse events, and bone remodeling of osseointegrated percutaneous implants for transhumeral amputees. Clin Orthop Relat Res 2014;472(10):2947–56.

15. Tillander J, Hagberg K, Berlin Ö, et al. Osteomyelitis risk in patients with transfemoral amputations treated with osseointegration prostheses. Clin Orthop Relat Res 2017;475(12):3100–8.

16. Leijendekkers RA, van Hinte G, Frölke JP, et al. Comparison of bone-anchored prostheses and socket prostheses for patients with a lower extremity amputation: a systematic review. Disabil Rehabil 2017;39(11):1045–58.

17. Al Muderis MM, Lu WY, Li JJ, et al. Clinically relevant outcome measures following limb osseointegration; systematic review of the literature. J Orthop Trauma 2018; 32(2):e64–75.

18. Coffey L, Gallagher P, Horgan O, et al. Psychosocial adjustment to diabetes-related lower limb amputation. Diabet Med 2009;26(10):1063–7.

19. Darnall BD, Ephraim P, Wegener ST, et al. Depressive symptoms and mental health service utilization among persons with limb loss: results of a national survey. Arch Phys Med Rehabil 2005;86(4):650–8.

20. Anderson D, Roubinov D, Turner A, et al. Perceived social support moderates the relationship between activities of daily living and depression after lower limb loss. Rehabil Psychol 2017;62(2):214–20.

21. Williams RM, Ehde DM, Smith DG, et al. A two-year longitudinal study of social support following amputation. Disabil Rehabil 2004;26(14–15):862–74.

22. Brier MJ, Williams RM, Turner AP, et al. Quality of relationships with caregivers, depression, and life satisfaction after dysvascular lower extremity amputation. Arch Phys Med Rehabil 2017;99(3):452–8.

23. Desmond D, Gallagher P, Henderson-Slater D, et al. Pain and psychosocial adjustment to lower limb amputation amongst prosthesis users. Prosthet Orthot Int 2008;32(2):244–52.

24. Chin T, Sawamura S, Fujita H, et al. Physical fitness of lower limb amputees. Am J Phys Med Rehabil 2002;81(5):321–5. Available at: http://www.ncbi.nlm.nih.gov/pubmed/11964571.

25. Yazicioglu K, Yavuz F, Goktepe AS, et al. Influence of adapted sports on quality of life and life satisfaction in sport participants and non-sport participants with physical disabilities. Disabil Health J 2012;5:249–53.

26. Laferrier JZ, Teodorski E, Cooper RA. Investigation of the impact of sports, exercise, and recreation participation on psychosocial outcomes in a population of veterans with disabilities: a cross-sectional study. Am J Phys Med Rehabil 2015;94(12):1026–34.

27. Wetterhahn KA, Hanson C, Levy CE. Effect of participation in physical activity on body image of amputees. Am J Phys Med Rehabil 2002;81(3):194–201.

28. Fatone S, Dillon M, Stine R, et al. Coronal plane socket stability during gait in persons with transfemoral amputation: pilot study. J Rehabil Res Dev 2014;51(8): 1217–28.

29. Fatone S, Caldwell R. Northwestern University flexible subischial vacuum socket for persons with transfemoral amputation-part 1: description of technique. Prosthet Orthot Int 2017;41(3):237–45.

30. Levy WS. Skin problems of the amputee. In: Bowker JH, Michael JW, editors. Atlas of limb prosthetics: surgical, prosthetic, and rehabilitation principles. 2nd edition. Rosemont (IL): American Academy of Orthopedic Surgeons; 1992. p. 681–8.

31. Morgan SJ, Mcdonald CL, Halsne EG, et al. Laboratory-and community-based health outcomes in people with transtibial amputation using crossover and energy-storing prosthetic feet: a randomized crossover trial. PLoS One 2018; 18. https://doi.org/10.1371/journal.pone.0189652.

32. McDonald CL, Kramer PA, Morgan SJ, et al. Energy expenditure in people with transtibial amputation walking with crossover and energy storing prosthetic feet: a randomized within-subject study. Gait Posture 2018;62:349–54.

33. Halsne EG, Mcdonald CL, Morgan SJ, et al. Assessment of low- and high-level task performance in people with transtibial amputation using crossover and energy-storing prosthetic feet: a pilot study. Prosthet Orthot Int 2018;1–9. https://doi.org/10.1177/0309364618774060.

34. Highsmith MJ, Kahle JT, Lura DJ, et al. Stair ascent and ramp gait training with the Genium knee. Tech Innov 2014;15(4):349–58.

35. Delussu AS, Brunelli S, Paradisi F, et al. Assessment of the effects of carbon fiber and bionic foot during overground and treadmill walking in transtibial amputees. Gait Posture 2013;38(4):876–82.

36. Gailey RS, Gaunaurd I, Agrawal V, et al. Application of self-report and performance-based outcome measures to determine functional differences between four categories of prosthetic feet. J Rehabil Res Dev 2012;49(4):597.

37. Ferris AE, Aldridge JM, Rábago CA, et al. Evaluation of a powered ankle-foot prosthetic system during walking. Arch Phys Med Rehabil 2012;93(11):1911–8.

38. Esposito ER, Whitehead JMA, Wilken JM. Step-to-step transition work during level and inclined walking using passive and powered ankle-foot prostheses. Prosthet Orthot Int 2016;40(3):311–9.

39. Herr HM, Grabowski AM. Bionic ankle-foot prosthesis normalizes walking gait for persons with leg amputation. Proc Biol Sci 2012;279(1728):457–64.

40. Grabowski AM, D'Andrea S. Effects of a powered ankle-foot prosthesis on kinetic loading of the unaffected leg during level-ground walking. J Neuroeng Rehabil 2013;10(1):49.

41. Zuo KJ, Olson JL. The evolution of functional hand replacement: from iron prostheses to hand transplantation. Plast Surg (Oakv) 2014;22(1):44–51.

42. Resnik L, Meucci MR, Lieberman-Klinger S, et al. Advanced upper limb prosthetic devices: implications for upper limb prosthetic rehabilitation. Arch Phys Med Rehabil 2012;93(4):710–7.

43. Fletchall S. Returning upper-extremity amputees to work. The O&P Edge. Northglenn (CO): Western Media LLC; 2005.

44. Hafner BJ. Clinical prescription and use of prosthetic foot and ankle mechanisms: a review of the literature. J Pediatr Ophthalmol 2005;17(4):S5–11.

45. Czerniecki JM. Research and clinical selection of foot-ankle systems. J Pediatr Ophthalmol 2005;17(4):S35–7.

Platelet-Rich Plasma Use in Musculoskeletal Disorders
Are the Factors Important in Standardization Well Understood?

Idris Amin, MD[a,b], Alfred C. Gellhorn, MD[b],*

KEYWORDS

- PRP Standardization • PRP Preparation • PRP Composition

KEY POINTS

- Currently, there is no standardization to the preparation and composition of platelet-rich plasma (PRP) for therapeutic use in musculoskeletal medicine, which may account for the variability in observed outcomes.
- Various classification systems have been proposed to measure and classify PRP composition, but none has been widely adopted.
- There are many different variables in the centrifugation process to create PRP, which can be optimized to produce the desired PRP product.

INTRODUCTION

Platelet-rich plasma (PRP) has received increased attention as a novel therapeutic treatment option of joint and tendon disease over the past 20 years. Although there is evidence of clinical effectiveness for osteoarthritis[1] and tendinopathy,[2] preparation methods are varied and the resultant PRP produced may have inconsistent results, from patient to patient, or even within the same patient on different days. A lack of standardization in production has been exacerbated by the proliferation of different kits from a variety of manufacturers. Recently, there has been a call to standardize how providers compare PRP, but additional research is needed to determine the optimal way to prepare PRP to achieve the best results. This article

Disclosure Statement: The authors have nothing to disclose.
[a] Department of Rehabilitation and Regenerative Medicine, Columbia University Medical Center, New York, NY, USA; [b] Department of Rehabilitation Medicine, Weill Cornell Medicine, 525 East 68th Street, Baker Pavilion F-1600, New York, NY 10065, USA
* Corresponding author.
E-mail address: alg9109@med.cornell.edu

discusses the most prevalent methodologies to prepare PRP, including an overview of the centrifugation process and a comparison of different preparation processes.

OVERVIEW OF PLATELET-RICH PLASMA

To appropriately recommend PRP to patients, providers must first have a thorough understanding of what the product is. PRP is defined as an autologous plasma product that has a concentration of platelets above baseline.[3,4] Given this simple definition, many different preparation methods, concentration levels, and product compositions all qualify as PRP. The resulting significant variability may help explain the inconsistent outcomes seen in the literature.[5,6] As of this writing, the Food and Drug Administration has approved PRP preparation systems for bone graft healing and for cutaneous wound management.[7] Preparation of PRP for use in joint and tendon disease is considered an off-label indication.

Growth Factors

It is believed that PRP works by facilitating the recruitment, proliferation, and maturation of factors that work in the healing cascade.[8] Recent studies indicate that the beneficial effects of PRP injections do not stem from the platelets themselves but rather the growth factors and proteins that are stored in the alpha-granules of platelets and that are released by activation of the platelets. Multiple studies suggest that the most influential growth factors are platelet-derived growth factor (PDGF), transforming growth factor ß (TGF-ß), vascular endothelial growth factor (VEGF), insulinlike growth factor, and epidermal growth factor.[9–14] PDGF, TGF-ß, and VEGF have been the most widely studied, and the presence of these factors in PRP mixtures is often used as a marker of a successful preparation.[10]

The growth factors are implicated in tissue repairing mechanisms, and counteract the effects of catabolic cytokines like tumor necrosis factor α (TNF-α) and interleukin 1 (IL-1).[15] They are also involved in modulating angiogenesis and protect endothelial cells from apoptosis, which helps ensure that adequate blood flow reaches the damaged tissue to initiate the wound healing process.[16] Specifically in degenerative joint diseases, growth factors play an important role in the regulation of articular cartilage and stimulate repair of damaged cartilage.[17]

Given that growth factors released from platelets are involved in the healing cascade for tendinopathic or intra-articular pathologies, it is important that the platelets are not activated prior to injection. Therefore, the viability and fragility of the platelets during the preparation process must be considered when creating the ideal preparation system.

Patient Selection

Because the recruitment of growth factors can mimic inflammatory pain, which sometimes worsens after the injection, physicians need to account for pain when selecting a patient for PRP injection. The pain from the injection itself can be limiting, especially in those that are aiming to return to activity or sport shortly after an intervention.

Another factor to consider when selecting patients for PRP injections is the serum platelet count prior to blood collection. Prior research suggests that for actual aggregation to occur, platelet counts need to be above $100,000/mm^3$.[18] Routine laboratory analysis with a complete blood cell count may be useful before preparing PRP to ensure patients do not have thrombocytopenia.

PLATELET-RICH PLASMA PREPARATION
Preparation Systems

The most common method in which PRP is prepared in the United States is through commercial kits that separate the blood product using a tabletop centrifuge system. There are many different commercial systems available on the market for PRP preparation, all with slight alterations in their preparation method.

Broadly speaking, most systems use either a single-spin or a double-spin preparation. In a single-spin preparation, the whole blood is centrifuged to create 3 basic components: the red blood cells collect at the bottom, a mixture of PRP and white blood cells in the middle, and platelet-poor plasma at the top. The spin time and rate of spin can vary, but the duration is generally under 10 minutes.[11] In a double-spin preparation, the whole blood product undergoes 2 spins through the centrifugation system. The first spin, also known as the hard spin, causes the red blood cells to settle at the bottom, a buffy coat of mainly white blood cells to form in the middle, and a layer of platelet plasma and some white blood cells to settle at the top. The second spin, also known as the soft spin, separates the PRP, which settles at the bottom of the tube with or without white blood cells, from the platelet-poor plasma.[19] Depending on the desired preparation, the buffy coat can be included in the second spin.[20] There is variation in the spin time and rate for double-spin systems as well, depending on the commercial system that is used.

There have been studies recently proposing cheaper alternatives for the preparation of PRP without the use of a commercial kit. This preparation consists of using a disposable 5-mL syringe modified to fit into a simple centrifugation machine, with the PRP settling near the tip of the syringe.[21] Although promising, the feasibility and safety of this method of PRP preparation remain unclear.

Classification Systems

With all of the different variations in the preparation of PRP, there have been several classification systems developed over the years to help compare and standardize the process. Mishra and colleagues[22] created a classification system that categorized PRP preparations based on the amount of platelets present, either 5 times above baseline or less than 5 times the baseline concentration, presence of white blood cells, and whether or not the platelets were activated. A few years later, Dohan Ehrenfest and colleagues[23] classified PRP based on the concentration of platelets and leukocytes and the presence or absence of fibrin. In 2012, Delong and colleagues[24] presented the platelet number, activation, white blood cell presence (PAW) classification system, which classified PRP based on platelet concentration, which ranged from baseline to above 1.2 million platelets/μL, activation of platelets, and the amount of white blood cells and neutrophils described as being above or below baseline. Finally, Mautner and colleagues[25] developed the platelet count, leukocyte presence, red blood cell presence, and use of activation (PLRA) classification system, which measured the absolute platelet concentration per microliter, concentration of leukocytes and neutrophils, red blood cell concentration, and activation by exogenous agents.

These classification systems, when used by the authors, have provided an increased amount of information about the PRP preparation used in clinical trials and provide a framework to assist in planning future PRP studies. Lack of a single agreed-on standard classification system continues to make comparison across studies difficult. Furthermore, given the rapid pace of development of PRP production techniques and equipment, existing classification systems need constant revision to address newer preparations. A summary of these classification systems is shown in **Table 1**.

Table 1	
Summary of classification systems for platelet-rich plasma preparations	
Classification System	**Dimensions Measured**
Mishra	• Amount of platelets present either 5 times above baseline or less than 5 times the baseline concentration • Presence of white blood cells • Activation of platelets
Dohan	• Concentration of platelets • Concentration of leukocytes • Presence or absence of fibrin
PAW	• Platelet concentration ranging from baseline to above 1.2 million platelets/μL • Activation of platelets • Amount of white blood cells and neutrophils described as above or below baseline
PLRA	• Absolute platelet concentration per microliter • Concentration of leukocytes and neutrophils • Red blood cell concentration • Activation by exogenous agents

Leukocyte-Rich Platelet-Rich Plasma Versus Leukocyte-Poor Platelet-Rich Plasma

As many recent classification systems have highlighted, the presence of leukocytes is an important dimension of the PRP mixture. Preparations of PRP can be categorized as leukocyte rich or leukocyte poor, and the presence of leukocytes often can be controlled through variables in the centrifugation process, including spin time, rate of spin, and number of spins.[26]

Several prior studies have analyzed the specific uses for leukocyte-rich and leukocyte-poor PRP. The general consensus is that leukocyte-rich preparations are better for muscle and tendon injuries, whereas leukocyte-poor preparations are more appropriate for intra-articular pathologies. Metcalf and colleagues[8] reported that leukocyte-rich PRP has proinflammatory cells that are beneficial for wound healing as well as treating tendinopathy. These proinflammatory cells are also believed a hindrance to chondrocyte repair after intra-articular injections. Braun and colleagues[27] found that leukocyte-rich PRP led to synovial cell death and the production of proinflammatory markers. Filardo and colleagues[28] reported increased side effects with the use of leukocyte-rich PRP for the treatment of osteoarthritis compared with leukocyte-poor preparations. Some providers believe, however, that the presence of leukocytes in PRP can be detrimental to the healing process in all types of pathologies, given that they induce a catabolic process that produces TNF-α and IL-1, which are the same factors that are believed targeted by the growth factors that are released by the platelets.[29]

CENTRIFUGATION PROCESS
Background on Centrifugation

Centrifugation processes are used to separate particles of a mixture into various homogenous layers. The earth's gravitational force can separate out particles that are suspended in a solution but this would take an exorbitant amount of time and is not feasible when considering clinical applications. The process is accelerated via centrifugation, which is defined as a method where a mixture is separated through spinning.

Particles are separated from a solution according to their size, shape, density, and speed of spin.[30] The overall viscosity of the solution that the particles are being separated from also can affect the centrifugation process. These principles help explain the variability in PRP mixture compositions.

To separate these particles, a centrifugal force is created and applied to the solution. The force (g), is calculated by the following equation: $g = mw^2r$, where m is the mass of the particle, w is the speed of the centrifuge in revolutions per minute, and r is the distance from the axis of the rotation to the particle.[30] For the purpose of PRP, the equation can also be defined as $g = (1.118 \times 10^{-5})S^2R$, where the constant is the mass of platelet, S is the speed of the centrifuge in revolutions per minute, and R is the radius of the rotor in centimeters.[31]

There are several variables within the PRP centrifugation process, including single spin versus double spin, the centrifugal force, time of spin, and other miscellaneous factors. The comparative impact of each of the factors here are elaborated on.

Single Spin Versus Double Spin

As discussed previously, PRP can be prepared via the single-spin or double-spin method of centrifugation. Initial studies looking at PRP used a single-spin system, which was believed to create a higher platelet count yield, approximately 2 times to 3 times above baseline.[11,32] When performing a second spin, Kahn and colleagues[32] found that platelet viability decreased, possibly due to lysing of the platelets during the centrifugation spin. More recent studies found that the double-spin method yielded a higher platelet concentration compared with single-spin preparations.[21] Additional studies are needed to explain the contradictory results in these studies.

Evidence also suggests that the pipetting process required to isolate the PRP from the solution can affect platelet counts and overall PRP composition.[33,34] Because single-spin methods require only 1 pipetting process rather than 2, human error is minimized, presenting an advantage of single-spin over double-spin preparations.

Although there have been several studies looking at the platelet count produced by single-spin or double-spin centrifugation, there is a dearth of research regarding the efficacy of the PRP produced by each method. Current belief is that a higher platelet count is more efficacious given that it has an increased concentration of growth factors present.[11,25,31]

Centrifugal Force

There is significant debate regarding the ideal centrifugal force for PRP preparation. Many of the commercially available kits range from 600 g to 2000 g, with the first spin often lower than the second spin in the double-spin system.[10] A survey of existing research presents contradictory findings on the optimal centrifugal force. Some studies have found that an increase in the force can lead to higher platelet concentrations.[21,35] Conversely, others found an inverse relationship between platelet counts and centrifugal force and that a higher g force can activate the platelets during the preparation process, instead of shortly after injection, which is believed more efficacious.[31,36–38] Sabarish and colleagues[39] incrementally increased the centrifugal force by increasing the speed of the spin and found a proportional decrease in platelet yield. Araki and colleagues[40] and Bausset and colleagues[41] advocated that the ideal centrifugation force is approximately 230 g to 270 g when using a double-spin preparation, with forces higher than this leading to a decreased platelet yield. Contrary evidence was presented, however, in a study by Dhurat and Sukesh,[31] who argued for a significantly higher centrifugal force of approximately 1000 g.

Finally, decreased centrifugal force was found to increase the number of leukocytes, in a single-spin PRP preparation study conducted by Choukroun and Ghanaati.[42] This is important for physicians to note when deliberately preparing leukocyte-rich PRP or leukocyte-poor PRP.

Duration of Spin

There is also a lack of consensus on the ideal amount of centrifuge time for PRP preparation. Perez and colleagues[38] found that longer spin time in a double-spin preparation increased platelet recovery and decreased the concentrations of white blood cells. Other studies found, however, that increased spin time led to decreased platelet count.[39,43,44] There is less known about the maximum time of centrifugation, but some providers are concerned that over-centrifugation can lead the platelets to discharge their growth factors prematurely.[21]

Miscellaneous Factors

There are several other factors in the centrifugation process that also affect the final composition of PRP. The temperature during the centrifugation process is important because it can affect platelet activation. Cooling of the preparation process is believed to prevent platelet activation, with the ideal temperature reported between 12°C and 16°C.[31,45] Many of the research studies aim to keep their PRP preparations at this temperature, but the temperature of the process with commercially available office kits has not been reported.[31]

When preparing PRP, there is a general consensus that the use of an anticoagulant is necessary because PRP cannot be centrifuged with clotted whole blood. The type of anticoagulant that is used remains a subject of debate, with most processes using ethylenediaminetetraacetic acid (EDTA) as opposed to citrate. EDTA has been found to produce more platelets but also is a stronger activator of PRP compared with citrate.[46,47] In addition, research indicates that EDTA can be more harmful than citrate to the PRP preparation because it has been shown to damage the platelets.[4,31,46]

Exogenous activation of the PRP solution prior to injection is another parameter to consider in the centrifugation process. PRP can be activated by calcium chloride, thrombin, or mechanical trauma.[31] Currently, the literature does not support preactivation prior to injection.[31,48]

During the centrifugation process, whole blood can be placed in a hard or a soft container. The common perception is that when the blood product hits the hard surface of the container, the products, including the platelets, can be lysed. In addition, Dhurat and Sukesh[31] noted that mechanical trauma can occur from hard container centrifugation, thereby prematurely activating the platelets. There also are studies that showed a nearly 86% increase in platelet recovery with the use of a soft plastic bag during centrifugation.[40] Overall, in comparison to other factors in PRP preparation, the data on the most appropriate container to use during centrifugation are limited.

Comparison of the Different Platelet-Rich Plasma Centrifugation Processes

With all the different variables that need to be accounted for during PRP preparation, providers are often left with many questions regarding the best approach to centrifugation. There also are many different commercial centrifugation machines on the market, which complicates the process. Most importantly, there is no clear evidence available to guide providers on which process produces highly efficacious PRP.

One variable used to measure the quality of PRP is the concentration of platelets that are produced through centrifugation. **Table 2** summarizes the components of

Table 2
Common commercial platelet-rich plasma systems on the market

Commercial System	Platelet Concentration ($\times 10^3$ μL)	Leukocyte Concentration ($\times 10^3$ μL)	Centrifugation Force (g) (First Spin/Second Spin)	Total Spin Time (min)
ACP	500	<1	350	5
Cascade	600–2900	<1	1100/1450	21
GPS III	1000–60,000	15–52	1100	15
Magellan	600–1500	<1–20	610/1240	10
SmartPrep	800–2600	8–35	1250/1050	24

Total spin time shows the sum of the first spin and second spin for double-spin systems.
Adapted from Oudelaar BW, Peerbooms JC, Huis In 't Veld R, et al. Concentrations of blood components in commercial platelet-rich plasma separation systems: a review of the literature. Am J Sports Med 2018;14(5); with permission.

common commercially available PRP systems.[10] In addition, when looking for the levels of platelet growth factors, the highest levels were found with the SmartPrep and GPS III (Zimmer Biomet) systems and lowest with the ACP (Arthrex) and Cascade systems.[49–51]

The concentration of growth factors is another variable that can be measured for the quality of PRP. As discussed previously, the most influential growth factors for healing that are located within the alpha granules of platelets are PDGF, TGF-ß, and VEGF. The literature is inconsistent with the concentration of PDGF and TGF-ß that is produced through the different commercial PRP systems. Concentration of VEGF, however, tends to be higher in PRP produced by systems like GPS III, which have a higher concentration of platelets and leukocytes.[10]

Clinical Outcomes Related to Leukocyte-rich Platelet-Rich Plasma and Leukocyte-Poor Platelet-Rich Plasma

Although the research is limited on the different systems available on the market today, a recent meta-analysis found strong evidence that leukocyte-rich PRP improved outcomes in tendinopathy.[52] These findings support the use of a centrifugation system like GPS III, which produces a higher concentration of leukocytes, when treating muscle and tendon injuries.[10] Studies have also found that leukocyte-poor PRP is efficacious in the treatment of intra-articular conditions like knee osteoarthritis.[53] The ACP system was found to produce the lowest number of leukocytes during PRP preparation.[10] Because most practices are not able to justify the purchase of multiple centrifugation systems, providers must choose a centrifugation process that is most applicable to the pathology that they encounter most often. There are some systems available on the market, however, that allow providers to adjust spin variables to produce either leukocyte-rich PRP or leukocyte-poor PRP.

SUMMARY

PRP preparation has evolved significantly over the past 20 years. When PRP was initially prepared, the process involved a large-volume blood collection (450 mL) that was transported to a central laboratory for centrifugation.[13,54] As technology continued to advance, in-office kits were developed for easier preparation and administration. Patients now only have 30 mL to 60 mL of blood drawn, and preparation time is quicker. These benefits have to be balanced, however, with the increased cost of using disposable kits, which can cost several hundred dollars.

To tackle the high costs, some researchers have looked at moving back to the large centrifugation model.[39] As a practical example of this proposal, the authors of this article developed a PRP preparation process that uses a blood bank centrifugation system to create and administer PRP in a developing country.[55] Patients with knee osteoarthritis donate 1 unit of whole blood to donation centers. The blood bank centrifugation system separates the whole blood into packed red blood cells, fresh-frozen plasma, and leukocyte-poor PRP. While the packed red blood cells and fresh frozen plasma are stored for donation to hospitalized patients, the PRP is then injected back into the donor. The procedure is free of charge for the donor because the costs of the centrifugation process by the blood bank are deemed minimal. Although this model requires at least 2 visits over 2 consecutive days, longer than an in-office kit requires, it can be considered for use in economically burdened and resource-poor areas, where other treatment options are not available.

A key best practice that emerges from the existing research regarding the use of PRP is to choose the most appropriate preparation to suit the targeted pathology. Even with recent advances in understanding PRP, however, there are still many unknowns about the factors and process that make the treatment effective for musculoskeletal conditions. There are several variables that have to be considered and, as a result of variability, data on the efficacy of PRP in patients with musculoskeletal conditions are mixed. The authors suggest that future PRP studies pursue these lines of inquiry to determine the optimal PRP preparation, set a standard to evaluate different PRP mixtures and preparation methods, assess the true efficacy of PRP for various musculoskeletal conditions, and explore ways to potentially manage and reduce costs.

REFERENCES

1. Su K, Bai Y, Wang J, et al. Comparison of hyaluronic acid and PRP intra-articular injection with combined intra-articular and intraosseous PRP injections to treat patients with knee osteoarthritis. Clin Rheumatol 2018;37(5): 1341–50.

2. Chen X, Jones IA, Park C, et al. The efficacy of platelet-rich plasma on tendon and ligament healing: a systematic review and meta-analysis with bias assessment. Am J Sports Med 2017;2016(1). 363546517743746.

3. Nurden AT, Nurden P, Sanchez M, et al. Platelets and wound healing. Front Biosci 2008;13:3532–48.

4. Marx RE. Platelet-rich plasma (PRP): what is PRP and what is not PRP? Implant Dent 2001;10(4):225–8.

5. Zhang H-F, Wang C-G, Li H, et al. Intra-articular platelet-rich plasma versus hyaluronic acid in the treatment of knee osteoarthritis: a meta-analysis. Drug Des Devel Ther 2018;12:445–53.

6. Ye Y, Zhou X, Mao S, et al. Platelet rich plasma versus hyaluronic acid in patients with hip osteoarthritis: a meta-analysis of randomized controlled trials. Int J Surg 2018;53:279–87.

7. 2017 biological device application approvals. US Food & Drug Administration; 2018. Available at: https://www.fda.gov/BiologicsBloodVaccines/Development ApprovalProcess/BiologicalApprovalsbyYear/ucm547560.htm. Accessed June 14, 2018.

8. Metcalf KB, Mandelbaum BR, McIlwraith CW. Application of platelet-rich plasma to disorders of the knee joint. Cartilage 2013;4(4):295–312.

9. Akhundov K, Pietramaggiori G, Waselle L, et al. Development of a cost-effective method for platelet-rich plasma (PRP) preparation for topical wound healing. Ann Burns Fire Disasters 2012;25(4):207–13.

10. Oudelaar BW, Peerbooms JC, Huis In 't Veld R, et al. Concentrations of blood components in commercial platelet-rich plasma separation systems: a review of the literature. Am J Sports Med 2018;14(5). 036354651774611.

11. Anitua E. Plasma rich in growth factors: preliminary results of use in the preparation of future sites for implants. Int J Oral Maxillofac Implants 1999;14(4):529–35.

12. Carlson NE, Roach RB. Platelet-rich plasma: clinical applications in dentistry. J Am Dent Assoc 2002;133(10):1383–6.

13. Marx RE, Carlson ER, Eichstaedt RM, et al. Platelet-rich plasma: Growth factor enhancement for bone grafts. Oral Surg Oral Med Oral Pathol Oral Radiol Endod 1998;85(6):638–46.

14. Ogino Y, Ayukawa Y, Kukita T, et al. The contribution of platelet-derived growth factor, transforming growth factor-beta1, and insulin-like growth factor-I in platelet-rich plasma to the proliferation of osteoblast-like cells. Oral Surg Oral Med Oral Pathol Oral Radiol Endod 2006;101(6):724–9.

15. Laver L, Marom N, Dnyanesh L, et al. PRP for degenerative cartilage disease: a systematic review of clinical studies. Cartilage 2017;8(4):341–64.

16. Ferrari G, Cook BD, Terushkin V, et al. Transforming growth factor-beta 1 (TGF-beta1) induces angiogenesis through vascular endothelial growth factor (VEGF)-mediated apoptosis. J Cell Physiol 2009;219(2):449–58.

17. Ulrich-Vinther M, Maloney MD, Schwarz EM, et al. Articular cartilage biology. J Am Acad Orthop Surg 2003;11(6):421–30.

18. Lanzkowsky P, Lipton JM, Fish JD. Lanzkowsky's manual of pediatric hematology and oncology. Cambridge (MA): Elsevier; 2016. https://doi.org/10.1016/c2013-0-23320-1.

19. Sonnleitner D, Huemer P, Sullivan DY. A simplified technique for producing platelet-rich plasma and platelet concentrate for intraoral bone grafting techniques: a technical note. Int J Oral Maxillofac Implants 2000;15(6):879–82.

20. Perez AGM, Lana JFSD, Rodrigues AA, et al. Relevant aspects of centrifugation step in the preparation of platelet-rich plasma. ISRN Hematol 2014;2014(4): 176060–8.

21. Fukaya M, Ito A. A new economic method for preparing platelet-rich plasma. Plast Reconstr Surg Glob Open 2014;2(6):e162.

22. Mishra A, Harmon K, Woodall J, et al. Sports medicine applications of platelet rich plasma. Curr Pharm Biotechnol 2012;13(7):1185–95.

23. Dohan Ehrenfest DM, Rasmusson L, Albrektsson T. Classification of platelet concentrates: from pure platelet-rich plasma (P-PRP) to leucocyte- and platelet-rich fibrin (L-PRF). Trends Biotechnol 2009;27(3):158–67.

24. DeLong JM, Russell RP, Mazzocca AD. Platelet-rich plasma: the PAW classification system. Arthroscopy 2012;28(7):998–1009.

25. Mautner K, Malanga GA, Smith J, et al. A call for a standard classification system for future biologic research: the rationale for new PRP nomenclature. PM R 2015; 7(4 Suppl):S53–9.

26. de Melo BAG, Martins Shimojo AA, Marcelino Perez AG, et al. Distribution, recovery and concentration of platelets and leukocytes in L-PRP prepared by centrifugation. Colloids Surf B Biointerfaces 2018;161:288–95.

27. Braun HJ, Kim HJ, Chu CR, et al. The effect of platelet-rich plasma formulations and blood products on human synoviocytes: implications for intra-articular injury and therapy. Am J Sports Med 2014;42(5):1204–10.

28. Filardo G, Kon E, Pereira Ruiz MT, et al. Platelet-rich plasma intra-articular injections for cartilage degeneration and osteoarthritis: single- versus double-spinning approach. Knee Surg Sports Traumatol Arthrosc 2012;20(10):2082–91.

29. Zhou Y, Zhang J, Wu H, et al. The differential effects of leukocyte-containing and pure platelet-rich plasma (PRP) on tendon stem/progenitor cells - implications of PRP application for the clinical treatment of tendon injuries. Stem Cell Res Ther 2015;6:173.

30. Anderson NG. An introduction to particle separations in zonal centrifuges. Natl Cancer Inst Monogr 1966;21:9–39.

31. Dhurat R, Sukesh M. Principles and methods of preparation of platelet-rich plasma: a review and author's perspective. J Cutan Aesthet Surg 2014;7(4):189–97.

32. Kahn RA, Cossette I, Friedman LI. Optimum centrifugation conditions for the preparation of platelet and plasma products. Transfusion 1976;16(2):162–5.

33. Michelson AD. Flow cytometry: a clinical test of platelet function. Blood 1996;87(12):4925–36.

34. Schmitz G, Rothe G, Ruf A, et al. European Working Group on clinical cell analysis: consensus protocol for the flow cytometric characterisation of platelet function. Thromb Haemost 1998;79(5):885–96.

35. Man D, Plosker H, Winland-Brown JE. The use of autologous platelet-rich plasma (platelet gel) and autologous platelet-poor plasma (fibrin glue) in cosmetic surgery. Plast Reconstr Surg 2001;107(1):229–37 [discussion: 238–9].

36. Dugrillon A, Eichler H, Kern S, et al. Autologous concentrated platelet-rich plasma (cPRP) for local application in bone regeneration. Int J Oral Maxillofac Surg 2002;31(6):615–9.

37. Amable PR, Carias RBV, Teixeira MVT, et al. Platelet-rich plasma preparation for regenerative medicine: optimization and quantification of cytokines and growth factors. Stem Cell Res Ther 2013;4(3):67.

38. Perez AGM, Lana JFSD, Rodrigues AA, et al. Relevant aspects of centrifugation step in the preparation of platelet-rich plasma. ISRN Hematol 2014;2014:176060.

39. Sabarish R, Lavu V, Rao SR. A comparison of platelet count and enrichment percentages in the platelet rich plasma (PRP) obtained following preparation by three different methods. J Clin Diagn Res 2015;9(2):ZC10–2.

40. Araki J, Jona M, Eto H, et al. Optimized preparation method of platelet-concentrated plasma and noncoagulating platelet-derived factor concentrates: maximization of platelet concentration and removal of fibrinogen. Tissue Eng Part C Methods 2012;18(3):176–85.

41. Bausset O, Giraudo L, Veran J, et al. Formulation and storage of platelet-rich plasma homemade product. Biores Open Access 2012;1(3):115–23.

42. Choukroun J, Ghanaati S. Reduction of relative centrifugation force within injectable platelet-rich-fibrin (PRF) concentrates advances patients' own inflammatory cells, platelets and growth factors: the first introduction to the low speed centrifugation concept. Eur J Trauma Emerg Surg 2018;44(1):87–95.

43. Landesberg R, Roy M, Glickman RS. Quantification of growth factor levels using a simplified method of platelet-rich plasma gel preparation. J Oral Maxillofac Surg 2000;58(3):297–300.

44. Okuda K, Kawase T, Momose M, et al. Platelet-rich plasma contains high levels of platelet-derived growth factor and transforming growth factor-beta and modulates the proliferation of periodontally related cells in vitro. J Periodontol 2003;74(6):849–57.

45. Macey M, Azam U, McCarthy D, et al. Evaluation of the anticoagulants EDTA and citrate, theophylline, adenosine, and dipyridamole (CTAD) for assessing platelet activation on the ADVIA 120 hematology system. Clin Chem 2002;48(6 Pt 1): 891–9.
46. Efeoglu C, Akçay YD, Ertürk S. A modified method for preparing platelet-rich plasma: an experimental study. J Oral Maxillofac Surg 2004;62(11):1403–7.
47. do Amaral RJFC, da Silva NP, Haddad NF, et al. Platelet-rich plasma obtained with different anticoagulants and their effect on platelet numbers and mesenchymal stromal cells behavior in vitro. Stem Cells Int 2016;2016:7414036.
48. Gentile P, Cole JP, Cole MA, et al. Evaluation of not-activated and activated PRP in hair loss treatment: role of growth factor and cytokine concentrations obtained by different collection systems. Int J Mol Sci 2017;18(2):408.
49. Castillo TN, Pouliot MA, Kim HJ, et al. Comparison of growth factor and platelet concentration from commercial platelet-rich plasma separation systems. Am J Sports Med 2011;39(2):266–71.
50. Magalon J, Bausset O, Serratrice N, et al. Characterization and comparison of 5 platelet-rich plasma preparations in a single-donor model. Arthroscopy 2014; 30(5):629–38.
51. Leitner GC, Gruber R, Neumüller J, et al. Platelet content and growth factor release in platelet-rich plasma: a comparison of four different systems. Vox Sang 2006;91(2):135–9.
52. Fitzpatrick J, Bulsara M, Zheng MH. The effectiveness of platelet-rich plasma in the treatment of tendinopathy: a meta-analysis of randomized controlled clinical trials. Am J Sports Med 2017;45(1):226–33.
53. Simental-Mendía M, Vílchez-Cavazos JF, Peña-Martínez VM, et al. Leukocyte-poor platelet-rich plasma is more effective than the conventional therapy with acetaminophen for the treatment of early knee osteoarthritis. Arch Orthop Trauma Surg 2016;136(12):1723–32.
54. Whitman DH, Berry RL, Green DM. Platelet gel: an autologous alternative to fibrin glue with applications in oral and maxillofacial surgery. J Oral Maxillofac Surg 1997;55(11):1294–9.
55. Ngayomela et al. Initiation of a platelet rich plasma program to treat osteoarthritis and impact the limited blood supply in Tanzania. In press.

Internet-Connected Technology in the Home for Adaptive Living

Stephen Hampton, MD

KEYWORDS

- Smart home • Home automation • Adaptive living

KEY POINTS

- Although not the primary target, individuals with disabilities can use recently developed, more affordable home automation, or Smart Home, products to enhance independence.
- Internet-connected consumer devices can provide increased control of the home to those with physical disabilities and increased safety inside the home for those with cognitive disabilities.
- Given the popularity of early Smart Home general consumer devices, it is reasonable to expect ongoing development of devices and device categories that could further augment the independence of individuals with disabilities.

INTRODUCTION

Throughout the history of rehabilitation, clinicians have applied available technologies at the time to increase the independence of individuals with disabilities. Advances in adaptive technology have often been a by-product of development for other purposes. For example, the mass production of plastics starting in the mid-twentieth century allowed orthotists to create lightweight and more form-fitting versions of the previously metal and leather orthoses.[1,2]

"Smart home" or home automation technology has been long imagined and popularized in science fiction. In the 1960s animated television show, The Jetsons, meals were prepared and household chores were completed by various robots at the touch of a button by the human characters. Early iterations of interconnected home systems were typically proprietary and prohibitively expensive for the average consumer. Expense was an even greater concern when systems were developed to address specific physical impairments or activity limitations for individuals with disabilities.[3] In addition, such targeted systems often had limited functionality.

The author has nothing to disclose.
Department of Physical Medicine and Rehabilitation, University of Pennsylvania, Perelman School of Medicine, 1800 Lombard Street, 1st Floor, Philadelphia, PA 19146, USA
E-mail address: Stephen.hampton@uphs.upenn.edu

Phys Med Rehabil Clin N Am 30 (2019) 451–457
https://doi.org/10.1016/j.pmr.2018.12.004
1047-9651/19/© 2018 Elsevier Inc. All rights reserved.

In parallel with the rapid dissemination of smartphone and tablet technology throughout much of the globe, a large market has developed of internet-connected devices for use in the home. These devices bring new methods to control and customize the behavior of traditional home technology. For example, a "smart" lighting system might turn on lights in a room whenever a signal from a smartphone indicates arrival at home. Furthermore, communication between devices, including devices from different manufacturers, can create useful combinations. A single bedtime routine could be triggered that locks external doors, arms an alarm system, turns off lights, and sets an air conditioner to a desired temperature for sleep. As new products are introduced, they could be incorporated into these "smart" systems further enhancing the possibilities for control of the home.

Although often viewed as novelty or convenience items, interconnected home devices could meaningfully enhance the independence and safety of individuals with physical and/or cognitive impairments. This article highlights categories of currently available consumer devices with potential for application to adaptive living. Any specific devices are mentioned to elucidate a particular function and should not be construed as an endorsement of that product or manufacturer. The industry of home automation and "Internet of things" has become crowded with companies creating devices with similar capabilities. This article is not meant to be an exhaustive catalog of devices but instead to outline the ways in which these novel devices might augment more traditional approaches to maximizing function.

CONTENT
Control Methods

The manner in which desired behaviors are elicited is central to any home automation system. To be widely accessible, especially to individuals with disabilities, control of smart devices needs to be intuitive and familiar. Fortunately, advancement in the methods for interacting with these devices has reduced the technical complexity for the user. A schematic for how different smart home products might interact is found in **Fig. 1**.

Smartphone and tablet computers have become ubiquitous, especially within the United States. The collective hours spent interacting with these mobile screens is a testament to their central role in our lives. As of February 2018, an estimated 77%

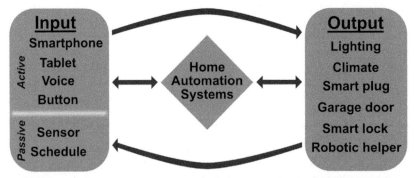

Fig. 1. Outline of home automation control methods and actions. Various active and passive control methods, or inputs, are used to trigger desired actions, or outputs, in connected devices. Commercial home automation systems have also been produced to integrate and coordinate the communication between multiple input and output home automation devices.

of Americans owned a smartphone, including 67% of those aged 54 to 72 and 30% of those aged 73 and older.[4,5]

Major manufactures of smartphones have developed software platforms that allow these devices to coordinate the actions of smart devices, such as Google Home, Apple HomeKit, and Amazon Alexa. Such platforms bring home automation to the same interfaces frequently used for checking email, reading news, and connecting with others via social media.

Through features built into smartphones and tablets and connections with third-party devices, even individuals unable to operate a touchscreen interface through traditional means can make use of smartphones. An individual with tetraplegia might use a tablet via signals from an electronic sip-and-puff controller. Once an adaptive approach for using smartphones and tablets is established, that individual has access to myriad abilities, including interaction with smart home technology.

Voice commands integrated into smartphones and dedicated products allows even those who have limited technical abilities a means of interacting with computer systems. As natural language processing has advanced, this conversation has become more fluid and less reliant on memorization of specific commands, furthering the general approachability. There has also been a steady growth in the actions achievable through verbal commands, although the possibilities are still fewer than those presented on screen interfaces. Voice command technology has particular salience for individuals with physical or visual limitations who may have previously found manipulation of a computer keyboard and mouse cumbersome. In addition, individuals with cognitive impairment may have difficulty remembering the steps to accomplish a desired task within a computer operating system, but may more readily learn to make spoken requests of a dedicated device. Unfortunately, this technology currently is not able to fully accommodate deficits in verbal communication, such as dysarthria or aphasia.

Passive sensors can be configured to trigger a variety of actions within a home without requiring direct human action. For example, if a monitor detects the temperature in a particular room rises above a desired range, it could send signals to turn on a ceiling fan and lower sun-blocking windows shades. These sensors might monitor for motion; opening of doors or windows; or internal conditions, such as temperature or humidity. These sensors connect with smart devices within the home to produce the desired action. Creating multistep rules for these actions increases the sophistication for what is possible, which may increase the chance that results are as desired. A sensor in a bedroom could be programmed to trigger lights to turn on when motion is detected in that room during specific daytime hours on specific days of the week, thus avoiding lights from turning on if one rolls in bed during sleep. Even if an individual was unable to interact with a smart system through other means, these passive sensors could provide her or him with increased control over a home's behavior.

Programmable physical buttons allow triggering of simple or complex smart home actions through a familiar mechanism. These buttons are mounted or moved anywhere within the home and may feature one or multiple physical buttons for producing actions. Unlike traditional buttons, these devices are setup to direct the behavior of multiple smart devices and reprogrammed to different purposes as needed. An individual with impairments in speech and fine motor control may have difficulty using voice commands or manipulating a smartphone, although they may be able to hit a button affixed to a wall, table, or wheelchair.

Connecting traditional devices to a home automation system is achieved through add-on adapters specific to that device or through smart electricity plugs. Many newer consumer products for the home feature an Internet connection and some are readily added into a smart home system. In some cases, this functionality is added on after the fact by products specific to that device, such as garage door openers or televisions. In others, Internet-connected electricity plugs can turn on or off power to devices based on rules or triggers from a home automation system. A bedtime routine might include providing power to a table fan and/or white noise machine with physical buttons left in the "on" position. These smart plugs can expand the available actions within a home automation system with existing electronics, potentially lower the cost required to develop such a system, and can allow inclusion of products that may not yet have commercially available versions with smart features.

Subsequent sections focus on specific functions of a smart home system that are triggered by the previously discussed control methods. Individuals with disabilities may benefit from smart technologies in the home if they are able to use one or a combination of the previously mentioned approaches. Continued advances in the mechanisms for directing the behavior of smart home systems and the menu of possible actions will likely further the potential for application to adaptive living.

Activities of Daily Living and Instrumental Activities of Daily Living

Basic functioning within rehabilitation literature is often described in terms of activities of daily living (ADL) and instrumental ADL (iADL). The ability to perform or to obtain necessary assistance to perform ADL and iADL is central for an individual to safely live in a community setting. Different forms of adaptive technology aim to support the performance of ADL and iADL and are selected based on an individual's impairments and limitations.

ADL are fundamental to self-care and include bathing, dressing, feeding, and mobility, among others.[6] Currently available commercial home automation technology is unlikely to directly enable someone who requires assistance with ADL to be more independent with these activities. Robotic caregivers hold promise in this area; however, they are not yet widely accessible within the commercial market and are thus beyond the scope of this article.

iADL are more complex tasks than ADL that remain important to function within the home and community.[6] Adaptive applications of current commercial home automation technology can more readily be identified within iADL. Examples within home management and safety maintenance are described next.

Comfort

Early commercial home automation devices have focused on comfort, specifically lighting and climate control. Although controlling the brightness level or color of lights in a room from one's smartphone is reasonably considered a novelty or convenience feature in most circumstances, allowing an individual, who cannot reach for a light switch, to turn lights on or off in a room could meaningfully enhance his or her quality of life. Smart lighting systems work through replacement of the light bulbs or the light switch with connected devices. Installation for the former is simpler, whereas the latter may be more cost effective depending on the number of light bulbs involved. Beyond possible impacts on independence, a smart lighting system with a motion sensor could ensure appropriate lighting in settings with increased risk of falls, such as during stair negotiation, and thus could impact the potential for injury within the home.

Smart thermostats and similar devices have allowed inclusion of climate control into home automation systems. Similar to smart lighting, these devices could enable an individual with a disability more direct input on conditions within the home. Such systems could also provide an early warning signal of malfunction, even to a caregiver outside the home, before an unsafe temperature is reached.

Safety and Security

A variety of Internet-connected devices have been developed for the purpose of safety and security. Many of these devices added an Internet connection to existing product categories, which in turn increased the options for interacting with these devices.

Connected security systems either add Internet connection to professionally installed systems or integrate a network of Internet-enabled sensor devices that are installed and expanded by the homeowner. In either case, an Internet connection could allow an individual with a disability expanded options for arming or disarming a security system. In addition, a caregiver could be provided with access to monitor a connected security system from a distance. Components of a security system often include sensors that can detect if a door or window is opened or if there is motion in a room. In addition to safety, these sensors could serve multiple home automation purposes, such as turning on entryway lights when a front door is opened.

Video doorbells provide a live or recorded view of an external entryway when a button is pressed. For individuals with mobility limitations, this could enhance their ability to interact with visitors and control access into their home. For example, after confirming the identity of an arriving caregiver on a smartphone screen, a connected smart lock could be unlocked using a voice command.

Smart locks expand the options for opening and securing a door. In addition to the traditional key, smart locks may open with numeric combinations; uniquely coded items that could be worn as bracelets; or control methods for other aspects of home automation, such as a voice command. Even if an individual is able to manipulate a key, having an alternate method available could decrease the effort required to enter and exit the home. A smart lock may also have the ability to send a reminder if left unlocked or simply lock itself after a set time interval. Increased control over access to one's home could be provided by smart locks, especially when combined with a video doorbell as described previously and depicted in **Fig. 2**.

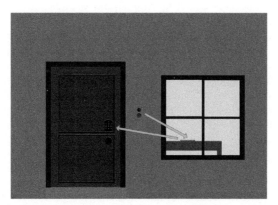

Fig. 2. Video doorbell and smart lock interacting with a tablet computer. Once activated, a video doorbell could allow an individual to quickly see and speak with a visitor through a tablet computer. If he or she wishes to allow this visitor to enter, a command could be sent through the same tablet computer to unlock a smart lock. In this way, an individual unable to move to an entryway door without assistance could independently verify and allow access to appropriate visitors.

Garage doors and gates with connection to the Internet provide another method for controlling access to a home. Similar to smart locks, these devices could send an alert if left unsecured or open. An individual with impairments in manual dexterity may find another home automation control method (eg, voice control) easier than a traditional garage door opener.

Robotic Assistants

The imagined robotic helpers of the Jetsons have begun to be realized in recent commercial products. These have included vacuums, mops, and lawn mowers capable of navigating through particular tasks on their own. Internet connection has been built into these products to allow communication with other elements of home automation including calling them into action by voice or at the push of a button. By integrating with a smart home system, these semiautonomous devices can assist with maintaining cleanliness and appearance of the home.

Robots capable of performing a variety of additional tasks, including more complex household activities, are under active development within the government, academia, and industry. As these are introduced into the commercial market in coming years, further potential applications to adaptive living should follow.

CONSIDERATIONS

Although some previously futuristic aspects of the Jetsons' household are now widely available as consumer products, others remain in the realm of developing technology or yet to be realized science fiction. Robotic involvement in more complex tasks within the home, such as caregiving, is primarily a research enterprise at this time. If robust robotic caregivers became an accessible reality, it would likely result in a significant decrease in the reliance of individuals with disabilities on assistance from other humans. Although the potential for benefit is great in this and other potential future advances in home automation, responsible adaptive application needs to contend with areas of concern, such as privacy and reliability.

Privacy is a common concern expressed in response to the expansion of electronic technology into ever more domains of life. This is especially relevant to home automation given the intimate data regarding daily life that is collected by such systems. A thorough discussion of the ethics surrounding technology and privacy is beyond the scope of this article, although a general awareness of this issue and common digital security pitfalls (eg, repeated use of an easily guessed password) may help in considering whether to bring a particular device into the home.

Reliability of devices to consistently perform as expected is essential for adaptive use. Although smart lights not turning on when expected may frustrate someone able to walk across a room to a wall switch, this occurring for an individual with limited mobility may result in abandonment of this adaptive device or worse an adverse event, such as a fall.

Evidence is currently limited regarding outcomes with use of commercial home automation, likely because of the novel and continuously evolving nature of these devices.[7] As in many other areas of rehabilitation, more study is needed to support decision-making in the application of this technology.

SUMMARY

Competition among commercial electronics companies has spurred rapid technologic advancement, the pace of which seems to be only accelerating. Once a cliché of science fiction, home automation technology has recently entered the mass market and increased the accessibility of such systems. Currently available devices seem most beneficial for certain iADL and advanced tasks. As Smart Home system continue to advance, there are likely to be additional applications for increasing independence of individuals with disabilities.

REFERENCES

1. Geyer R, Jambeck JR, Law KL. Production, use, and fate of all plastics ever made. Sci Adv 2017;3:e1700782.
2. Bensman AS, Lossing W. A new ankle-foot orthosis combining the advantages of metal and plastics. Orthotics and Prosthetics 1979;33:3–10.
3. Steel EJ, Buchanan R, Layton N, et al. Currency and competence of occupational therapists and consumers with rapidly changing technology. Occup Ther Int 2017; 2017:5612843.
4. Demographics of mobile device ownership and adoption in the United States. Pew Research Center Internet & Technology. Available at: http://www.pewinternet.org/fact-sheet/mobile/ Accessed July 27, 2018.
5. Millennials stand out for their technology use. Pew Research Center Internet & Technology. Available at: http://www.pewresearch.org/fact-tank/2018/05/02/millennials-stand-out-for-their-technology-use-but-older-generations-also-embrace-digital-life/ Accessed July 27, 2018.
6. Occupational therapy practice framework: domain and process (3rd edition). Am J Occup Ther 2014;68:S1–48.
7. Martin S, Kelly G, Kernohan WG, et al. Smart home technologies for health and social care support. Cochrane Database Syst Rev 2008;(3):CD006412.

Data Science in Physical Medicine and Rehabilitation
Opportunities and Challenges

Kenneth J. Ottenbacher, PhD, OTR[a],*, James E. Graham, PhD, DC[b],
Steve R. Fisher, PT, PhD, GCS[c]

KEYWORDS

- Data science • Big data • Data networks • Rehabilitation science • Outcomes

KEY POINTS

- Data science represents a new approach to developing knowledge in biomedical research.
- Data science is producing innovative ways to acquire, store, analyze, and interpret large amounts of diverse medical and health-related information.
- The implementation of data science will enhance the ability of physical medicine and rehabilitation to reduce disability and improve health care services and outcomes.

INTRODUCTION

Using data to drive discovery has been a hallmark of scientific investigation since the 1600s, beginning with the writings of Sir Francis Bacon regarding the modern scientific method.[1] From its earliest days, the goal of data-driven health science has been to understand the human body and improve human health and well-being. The biomedical scientific community is currently experiencing a dramatic expansion in how data are being used to generate new knowledge and accomplish the goals of reducing disease and disability and improving health care delivery.[2]

In 2011, a special issue of *Science* predicted that big data, made possible by enormous new sources of data, would sweep through academia, business, health care, and government. The authors argued there was no area that would remain untouched.[3] Several factors have contributed to this data expansion. Advances in computing and information technology, biostatistics, bioinformatics, internet capacity,

Disclosure Statement: The authors were supported by grants K12 HD055929 and P2CHD065702 from the National Institutes of Health.
[a] Division of Rehabilitation Sciences, University of Texas Medical Branch, 301 University Boulevard, Route 1137, Galveston, TX 77555-1137, USA; [b] Department of Occupational Therapy, Center for Community Partnerships, Colorado State University, 320 Occupational Therapy Building, Fort Collins, CO 80523-1573, USA; [c] Department of Physical Therapy, University of Texas Medical Branch, 301 University Boulevard, Route 1144, Galveston, TX 77555-1144, USA
* Corresponding author.
E-mail address: kottenba@utmb.edu

Phys Med Rehabil Clin N Am 30 (2019) 459–471
https://doi.org/10.1016/j.pmr.2018.12.003
1047-9651/19/© 2018 The Authors. Published by Elsevier Inc. This is an open access article under the CC BY-NC-ND license (http://creativecommons.org/licenses/by-nc-nd/4.0/).

and cloud technology have made it possible to digitally analyze, store, transfer, and share large datasets at levels that were not imagined a few years ago.

These changes have resulted in the emergence of a new scientific and academic discipline referred to as data science. The National Institutes of Health (NIH) recently released their Strategic Plan for Data Science.[4] The NIH plan defines data science as an "interdisciplinary field of inquiry in which quantitative and analytical approaches, processes, and systems are developed and used to extract knowledge and insights from increasingly large and/or complex sets of data."[4(p29)] **Box 1** includes the broad components of the NIH Strategic Plan for Data Science.

DATA SCIENCE AND BIG DATA

The terminology in data science can be confusing. Data science involves using computer-based systems and processes to analyze large amounts of data and extract knowledge from them.[5] In medicine and health care, data science is often described in combination with big data and the NIH Big Data to Knowledge (BD2K) program.[2,6] The BD2K program is a trans-NIH initiative created in 2012 to support the research and development of innovative and transformative quantitative approaches and tools to maximize and accelerate the integration of big data into biomedical research.[2,6] The NIH introduced a variety of funding and research capacity building methods and opportunities for big data in conjunction with the BD2K program.

DATA SCIENCE AND REHABILITATION

Data science and big data are new areas to physical medicine and rehabilitation with important implications for practice and research. Data science also poses challenges involving building research capacity and expanding the traditional scientific culture within physical medicine and rehabilitation and rehabilitation science. Clinicians and investigators involved in rehabilitation research are trained in professional and graduate programs that focus on conducting prospective, patient-oriented clinical research, often emphasizing clinical trials. The resulting studies frequently involve

---

Box 1
Components and activities associated with the National Institutes of Health Strategic Plan for Data Sciences

Data Infrastructure	Modernized Data Ecosystem	Data Analytics and Management Tools	Workforce Development	Stewardship and Sustainability
• Optimize data storage and security • Connect NIH data systems	• Modernize data repository ecosystem • Support storage and sharing of individual datasets • Better integrate clinical and observational data into biomedical data science	• Support useful, generalizable, and accessible tools and workflows • Broaden utility and access to specialized tools • Improve discovery and cataloguing resources	• Enhance NIH data-science workforce • Expand the National research workforce • Engage a broader community	• Develop policies for a FAIR data ecosystem • Enhance stewardship

Abbreviation: FAIR, Findable, Accessible, Interoperable, Reusable.

Adapted from NIH Strategic Plan for Data Science. 2018. Available at: https://datascience.nih.gov/strategicplan. Accessed July 20, 2018; with permission. FAIR, Findable, Accessible, Interoperable, Reusable.

small samples and are located in 1 setting. This model of training produces rehabilitation scientists who are not familiar with the methods, analytical procedures, and interpretation of big data; or with the application of data science procedures involving substantial amounts of information, often collected from multiple settings, over long periods of time, and including a large number of variables.

Paradigm shifts in health care have become the norm. Twenty years ago, translational research was in its infancy. Now, it is the core concept underpinning research in medical practice and health outcomes. Ten years ago the idea of patient-centered outcomes research was just being introduced. Now, actively including stakeholders in the research process is the rule rather than the exception. Similarly, qualitative research was long considered by many as soft science. Today, mixed methods are viewed as a powerful approach in studying human health. The recent emergence of big data and data science likely portend the next series of transformative changes. Segal and colleagues[7] outlined the process for identifying core competencies the clinical research workforce should acquire when pursuing new research standards. Their focus is on comparative effectiveness research, but the principles apply to big data and data science also.

The purpose of this article is to introduce readers with backgrounds in physical medicine and rehabilitation and rehabilitation science to methods and approaches used in data science. The information presented in the remainder of this article is not meant to be inclusive of the topics and methods involved in data science. The areas discussed include

- Big data and large data – definitions and applications relevant to physical medicine and rehabilitation
- Data sharing – the development of data warehouses and the requirements to share data from completed studies and the opportunities they provide in rehabilitation
- Resources – descriptions of programs and activities helping to build research capacity in data science
- Implications – identify opportunities in physical medicine and rehabilitation for applying data science

BIG DATA

As noted previously, big data in biomedical and health research have been defined and popularized by the BD2K program. The NIH describes the BD2K program as having 2 phases.[8,9] Phase 1, from 2012 to 2017, comprised a period of raising awareness, defining parameters, and developing infrastructure. The programs developed during this period were designed to promote the understanding and broad use of biomedical big data. The funding efforts in Phase 1 focused on creating and disseminating software and analytical methods that could be used across wide areas of biomedical research. BD2K Centers of Excellence were established to promote awareness and build research capacity by funding a variety of research and dissemination projects. Phase 2 of BD2K began in 2018 and is scheduled to continue through 2021. The purpose of Phase 2 is to promote the projects and products developed in Phase 1 and make them available to members of the biomedical research community. Another important goal of Phase 2 is to integrate the BD2K program and products into the NIH strategic plan related to the expanding domain of data science.[8]

Definitions

This section includes a brief description of the distinction between big data and large data as defined and used throughout the remainder of this article. There is no universally accepted definition of big data. Big data are generally defined as including datasets with sizes beyond the ability of traditional software tools to capture, clean, manage, and process the information within a reasonable time-period.[2,6] Big data analysis involves new methods and technologies (eg, example, machine learning) that require new forms of software and the integration of data that are diverse, complex, and exist on a massive scale.[2,6]

Roski and colleagues[10] make a distinction between big data and large data based on the size and type of data analyzed and the complexity of the analyses (**Fig. 1**). An example of big data related to rehabilitation is the Mobilize Center, an NIH BD2K Center of Excellence that is using modern data science tools to integrate and analyze information from a range of wearable sensors, smartphones, and other personal electronic devices used in homes, the community, clinics, and research centers around the world to better understand and improve human mobility.[11] The Mobilize Center is currently focusing on 3 areas: cerebral palsy management, gait rehabilitation research, and weight monitoring and control through physical activity. This combination of different topic areas and target populations, along with a wide range of wearable sensors and data formats, is characteristic of big data analytics as presented in **Fig. 1**. In contrast, a large data study might include using millions of Medicare claims files to study a health outcome (eg, hospital readmission). Such a research project involves a large number of patient records. However, the data are of the same type (eg, Medicare claims files), focus on 1 outcome (hospital readmission),[12] and could be analyzed using traditional statistical procedures. Such a study would be included in the large data analytics cell (see **Fig. 1**).

Both big data and large data approaches qualify as data science as discussed previously and defined in the NIH Strategic Plan.[4] Big data and large data studies are not

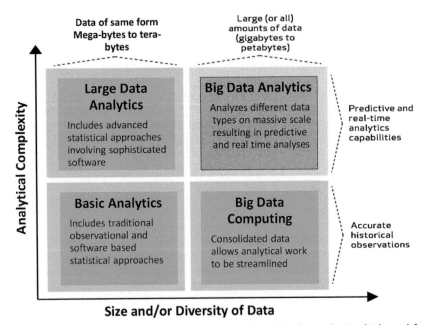

Fig. 1. Data analytical approach by size of data and analytical complexity. (*Adapted from* Roski J, Bo-Lin GW, Andrews TA. Creating value in health care through big data: opportunities and policy implications. Health Aff 2014;33(7):1120; with permission.)

commonly reported in the physical medicine and rehabilitation literature. A recent study showed that in 2 separate rehabilitation journals, cross-sectional clinical trials were the most common research design.[13] The classification category most likely to include large or big data studies in this article was labeled as cohort studies. The number of cohort studies reported in both rehabilitation journals remained stable from 2005 to 2015, at about 15%.[13] Examination of the cohort design studies published from 2012 to 2015 in the 2 rehabilitation journals revealed that less than 10% of the studies included sample sizes greater than 100, indicating that few studies were published during this period that would qualify as involving large or big data.

DATA SCIENCE OPPORTUNITIES

In this section are examples of several data resources that involve large or big data and illustrate the scope of data science. The data and material contained in these programs include information relevant to important clinical, scientific, and policy questions in physical medicine and rehabilitation.

The Affordable Care Act and Health Care Reform

The implementation of the Affordable Care Act is producing changes in the delivery of health care.[14] These changes have potentially far-reaching implications. Examples relevant to physical medicine and rehabilitation include changes in the health care payment system from fee-for-service to a model based on bundled payment and the introduction of national quality measures to improve outcomes. Bundled payment aggregates projected costs for several services over time into a single reimbursement for an episode of care and is designed to facilitate collaboration among providers and incentivize quality. These changes are resulting in the creation of new large datasets within Medicare and private health care systems designed to measure the value of patient care instead of the volume of services and procedures provided.[15]

The Improving Medicare Post-Acute Care Transformation Act of 2014 (IMPACT Act)[16] is another component of health care reform that is generating large amounts of data related to rehabilitation. The act requires the submission of standardized data by long-term care hospitals (LTCHs), skilled nursing facilities (SNFs), home health agencies (HHAs), and inpatient rehabilitation facilities (IRFs). The IMPACT Act will result in the development and implementation of quality measures in areas such as functional status, cognitive function, skin integrity, falls, and discharge to the community that will influence the future of postacute rehabilitation service delivery.[16,17]

Data Warehouses Relevant to Rehabilitation and Disability

Hospital mergers, health system expansions, and federal requirements for developing and implementing new payment systems and quality measures are resulting in the creation of private, commercial, and federal data warehouses and repositories.[18] Examples include data warehouses such as MarketScan, Clinometrics, and OPTUM. These data warehouses contain electronic health records (EHRs) and patient-level information that can be used to develop patient management and evaluation programs across large health systems or individual health care facilities. Information from these data warehouses and repositories are being used by data scientists. Some repositories include the archived research findings and data from previously conducted research investigations. The Data and Specimen Hub (DASH) supported by the National Institute for Child Health and Human Development (NICHD) at the NIH is an example of a repository containing information and original data from studies funded by the

NICHD. These archived data are available for secondary data analyses by other investigators.[19] The DASH is described in more detail below.

Data warehouses and repositories represent a valuable resource to monitor and evaluate existing and new programs in ways that have not been possible in the past. Several studies examining a specific intervention or similar outcome measures could be combined and integrated to explore new questions not considered in the original studies. Data science skills and expertise will be required to access, analyze, and interpret the information included in data warehouses and repositories.

Data Networks – Patient-Centered Outcomes Research National Network

The Patient-Centered Outcomes National Network (PCORnet) is a national network supported by the Patient-Centered Outcomes Research Institute[20] (**Box 2**). The network includes a consortium of hospitals, health systems, clinics, and patient partnerships. The PCORnet represents over 100 million participants. The data resources component of PCORnet is available to investigators through the PCORnet Front Door. PCORnet provides workshops and training programs where data scientist and clinical investigative teams can learn how to develop proposals and request PCORnet data.[20] Learning basic skills in data science is part of this process.

Data Networks – National Institutes of Health All of Us Program

The All of Us program is a key element of the NIH Precision Medicine Initiative.[21] The All of Us research program is an effort by the NIH to gather data over many years from one million people living in the United States, with the ultimate goal of accelerating research and improving health. Unlike research studies that are focused on a specific disease or population, All of Us is designed to serve as a national research resource to inform a range of studies covering a variety of health conditions (**Box 3**). The data will be collected by the NIH from volunteer participants.[21] Deidentified data will be available to investigators to conduct studies designed to better understand the disease process at the patient level in ways only possible using a large cohort with data collected over time. The protocol for data collection is being developed by the NIH.[21] The All of Us program represents a unique opportunity for physical medicine and rehabilitation investigators and data scientists.

The examples presented are meant to illustrate the type and variety of resources and opportunities emerging in the rapidly expanding world of data science relevant to physical medicine and rehabilitation. The overall impact of data science on health care and biomedical research is beyond the scope of this article. The NIH Strategic

---

Box 2
The Patient-Centered Outcomes Research National Network

- PCORnet is an initiative funded by the Patient-Centered Outcomes Research Institute (PCORI).

- PCORnet is a national "network of networks" that collects data routinely gathered in a variety of health care settings, including hospitals, doctors' offices, and community clinics.

- Its primary purpose is to facilitate potential investigators, patient groups, health care organizations, clinicians, and industry scientists to leverage PCORnet's infrastructure and collaborate on patient-centered clinical research.

Adapted from PCORnet: National Patient-Centered Clinical Research Network. Available at: http://www.pcornet.org/. Accessed June 22, 2018; with permission.

Box 3
Core values of the All of Us Research Program

A set of core values guide the development and implementation of the All of Us Research Program:
- Participation is open to all.
- Participants reflect the rich diversity of the United States.
- Participants are partners.
- Participants have access to their information.
- Data will be accessed broadly for research purposes.
- Security and privacy will be of highest importance.
- The program will be a catalyst for positive change in research.

Adapted from National Institutes of Health. The All of Us Research Program. U.S. Department of Health and Human Services. Available at: https://allofus.nih.gov/. Accessed June 15, 2018; with permission

---

Plan for Data Science released in June 2018 provides an overview of potential opportunities.[4] One component of data science with particular relevance for clinicians and investigators in physical medicine and rehabilitation is the development of guidelines and policies associated with data sharing and secondary analyses of existing research data related to rehabilitation and disability.

DATA SHARING AND DATA SCIENCE

In 2013, the White House Office of Science and Technology Policy published a report entitled Increasing Access to the Results of Federally Funded Scientific Research.[22] The report includes a mandate that all federal agencies funding more than $100 million in research or development projects annually must develop policies and procedures to make the results, information, and data generated by the research available to the public, industry, and the scientific community. A National Academies of Sciences report published in 2015 contains recommendations and procedures to help make the results and data from clinical trials and related clinical research available for dissemination and sharing.[23]

This is a topic that is poorly understood by many investigators. It is of particular importance to rehabilitation science and physical medicine and rehabilitation because there is a focus in the federal data-sharing requirements on clinical research. In a viewpoint article in *The Journal of the American Medical Association*, Ross and Krumholz write, "Momentum is gaining toward open science through data sharing. The imperative is to find successful pathways to share data that are attentive to all stakeholders, yet serve the best interest of society. The full potential of the clinical research enterprise can be realized by creating a culture that promotes data sharing and provides credit to those who do – and consequences to those who do not."[24]

Developing a "culture that promotes data sharing" in physical medicine and rehabilitation is in the very early stages. In an editorial titled Open and Abundant Data is the Future of Rehabilitation and Research, Babbage[25] reviews the 2013 US government requirement that data resulting from federally funded research be "made openly available in machine-readable formats."[25] He goes on to note that few studies in rehabilitation are ready to meet the federal requirements and that significant opportunities and challenges lie ahead. Babbage argues that rehabilitation researchers need to develop strategies to address the mandate and take advantage of the research opportunities it presents.[25] These opportunities will require data management and analytical skills not widely used in physical medicine and rehabilitation research.

Sharing research data is widely acknowledged as a sensible and cost-effective means for translating findings from federally funded research into knowledge and practice to improve health.[22,26] Making previously collected data available to consumers, providers, researchers, and policy makers has many benefits, including decreased redundancy, adding new perspectives from other disciplines, replication of the findings with more modern analytical techniques, merging data from smaller studies into larger datasets with greater statistical power, and practical opportunities for comparative effectiveness research. There are challenges also, including data management and storage, controlling access, maintaining scientific integrity, and complying with Health Insurance Portability and Accountability Act of 1996 (HIPAA) confidentiality and privacy concerns.[27,28]

Federal agencies supporting biomedical research are developing programs to meet the White House Office of Science and Technology requirement.[22] The National Science Foundation (NSF) has established a Dissemination and Data Sharing Policy.[29] The Agency for Healthcare Research and Quality (AHRQ) has a detailed plan and protocol for public access and sharing of funded research data supported by the AHRQ.[30]

The National Center for Medical Rehabilitation Research (NCMRR) is housed in the NICHD. Thus, rehabilitation and disability researchers funded through the NCMRR are encouraged to use the DASH repository introduced previously. The DASH repository enables NICHD-funded investigators to organize and store data from their research studies. These data can be used for secondary data analyses and related research activities by other investigators, if appropriate criteria are meet.[19] DASH currently includes approximately 90 archived datasets. To access the data and related information, users are required to register and to complete a data use agreement. Detailed information is available on the DASH Web site.[19] Obviously, 90 studies represents a small portion of the research funded by the NICHD. At this time, no timeline for mandatory participation of NICHD-funded investigators in DASH has been established. Different institutes within the NIH are developing various strategies and approaches to meet the data dissemination and sharing requirements issued by the White House Office of Science and Technology Policy.[22]

Other research-related data repositories represent partnerships among federal agencies based on topics or populations. The Federal Interagency for Traumatic Brain Injury Research (FITBIR) was developed as a collaboration involving over 20 NIH institutes and federal departments with research and clinical interest in TBI.[31] The goal of FITBIR is to share data across the entire field of TBI research in order to facilitate collaboration between centers and laboratories and promote interconnectivity with other informatics platforms. Participants in FITBIR share methodologies and research tools that allow secondary data analyses, as well as aggregation, integration, and comparisons using the contributed data[31] (**Box 4**).

In establishing the NIH Strategic Plan for Data Science,[4] the following data-sharing implementation strategies have been proposed: store data efficiently and securely; make data usable to as many people as possible; develop a research workforce to advance data science; and set policies for productive, efficient, secure, and ethical data use. These objectives are referred to in the strategic plan as the FAIR principles. FAIR stands for Findable, Accessible, Interoperable, and Reusable[4,32] (**Box 5**).

Given the rise in the number of data repositories warehousing research datasets, there are now data search engines for discovering topic-specific datasets and larger data repositories. The biomedical and healthCAre Data Discovery Index Ecosystem (bioCADDIE) is a leading entity in this new domain. With BD2K funding, bioCADDIE developed a biomedical research data search engine called DataMed.[33] As of August, 2018, DataMed had indexed 75 repositories and more than 2.3 million datasets. This is

---

Box 4
The federal interagency for traumatic brain injury research

The FITBIR Informatics System is an extensible, scalable informatics platform for TBI relevant data (eg, medical imaging, clinical assessment, environmental and behavioral history) and for all data types (eg, text, numeric, image, time series). FITBIR was developed to share data across the entire TBI research field and to facilitate collaboration between laboratories, as well as interconnectivity with other informatics platforms. Sharing data, methodologies, and associated tools, rather than summaries or interpretations of this information, can accelerate research progress by allowing repeat analysis of data, as well as repeat aggregation, integration, and rigorous comparison with other data, tools, and methods. This community-wide sharing requires common data definitions, standards and comprehensive, coherent informatics approaches.

From Federal Interagency Traumatic Brain Injury Research (FITBIR) Informatics System. Available at: https://fitbir.nih.gov/. Accessed May 23, 2018; with permission.

---

a global initiative covering all research fields. However, with selective searching and a transdisciplinary approach, DataMed can be a useful resource for complementing and expanding rehabilitation research programs and opportunities.

As the NIH Strategic Plan for Data Science is implemented, there will be modifications and efforts to standardize the data-sharing plans and programs across the NIH institutes and centers, including those described previously. The opportunities for data sharing and obtaining access to the information contained in studies funded by federal research dollars represent a unique and important opportunity for the field of physical medicine and rehabilitation. The following section describes some rehabilitation-specific resources available to help members of the rehabilitation sciences and physical medicine and rehabilitation community take advantage of the opportunities and address the challenges associated with data science.

DATA SCIENCE RESOURCE FOR PHYSICAL MEDICINE AND REHABILITATION

The Center for Large Data Research and Data Sharing in Rehabilitation (CLDR)[34] is an NIH-funded consortium including the University of Texas Medical Branch, Cornell

---

Box 5
Guiding principles of the National Institutes of Health's strategic plan for data science

FAIR guiding principles
  Findable
- Data are assigned a unique identifier.
- Data are described in detail.
- Data are registered or indexed in a searchable resource.
  Accessible
- Data are retrievable using a standardized protocol.
- The protocol is open, free, and universally available.
- The protocol allows for authentication and authorization when necessary.
  Interoperable
- Data use a formal, accessible, shared, and widely used language/software.
- Data use vocabularies that follow FAIR principles.
- Data include qualified references to other data.
  Reusable
- Data are richly described with accurate attributes.
- Data are released with a clear and accessible data usage license.
- Data meet domain-relevant community standards.

Box 6
Activities of the Center For Large Data Research and Data Sharing in Rehabilitation

Education and Training	Data Directory	Data Sharing	Pilot Projects	Visiting Scholars
Workshops, on-line seminars and training modules to develop skills in large data research and data sharing	Listing of available datasets including purpose, variables, access, and contact information	Support for linking/merging and archiving data from completed rehabilitation studies to promote secondary data analyses	Collaborative projects with CLDR mentors/ investigators using large data related to rehabilitation and recovery	Collaborate with CLDR mentors using large rehabilitation datasets or archived data; appointed up to 6 months

Adapted from Center for Large Data Research and Data Sharing in Rehabilitation. University of Texas Medical Branch. Available at: https://www.utmb.edu/cldr. Accessed June 21, 2018; with permission.

University, University of Michigan-Ann Arbor, and Colorado State University. The center began operation in 2010 with the goal of building scientific capacity by increasing the quantity and quality of rehabilitation research using large complex datasets. The center was funded again in 2015, and the objectives were expanded to include a focus on data sharing and secondary analyses of archived data. The objectives of the center are to: raise awareness of research opportunities in data science; teach and disseminate skills necessary to conduct research related to large data and data sharing; provide in-person and small group training in data science; support pilot studies involving large data, big data, and the use of archived data (data sharing); and develop interdisciplinary collaborations in data science.

The activities and services supported and provided by the center are presented in **Box 6**.

Examples of the center's programs with information and how to apply for the pilot project funding, education and training activities, and visiting scholar program can be found on the center's Web site.[34]

The center is part of the Rehabilitation Research Resource Network[35] supported by the NIH. The network includes 6 centers providing scientific support and resources to rehabilitation investigators and clinicians across the country. Information about the network topic areas and services is available on the Rehabilitation Research Resource Network Web site.[35] It is important to understand that the purpose of these centers is not to conduct primary research. Rather, their mission is to provide scientific infrastructure including services similar to those in **Box 6** (eg, pilot studies) and to build research capacity in areas important to physical medicine and rehabilitation.

SUMMARY

The clinical and scientific impacts of big data and the developing field of data science on physical medicine and rehabilitation are impossible to predict. There will be an impact. There will also be opportunities and challenges. Creating strategies to take advantage of the opportunities and minimize the challenges is important for the future of physical medicine and rehabilitation.

Disability in America, published by the National Academies in 1991,[36] contributed to the Americans with Disabilities Act and raised national awareness of disability and rehabilitation. In spite of the increased visibility created by Disability in America, many of the report's recommendations were not addressed. Relevant to this article is recommendation 6, which proposed establishing a program of population-based research to create a national disability surveillance system. The intent was to create a nationwide database that would be updated regularly. The database would provide the ability to monitor the prevalence and incidence of disability in the United States. In addition to monitoring the prevalence and incidence of disability over time, and in different parts of the country, the surveillance system would also track causal phenomenon, risk factors, functional status, and quality of life. This information would be essential in planning prevention and intervention programs and guiding the allocation of resources.

Follow-up reports from the National Academies were published in 1997 and 2007.[37,38] These reports examined the status of past recommendations and identified new priorities. The Future of Disability in America, published in 2007, states "The lack of a comprehensive disability monitoring program, highlighted in the 1991 IOM report, remains a serious shortcoming in the nation's health statistics system. Today, disability statistics must be patched together from multiple, often inconsistent, surveys... overall, monitoring efforts continue to fall short of providing the nation with the basic data that it needs to monitor disability and manage the future."[39(p5)]

The advent of big data and the development of data science provide the ability to address this, and other recommendations from the National Academies' reports.[36–38] Successfully addressing recommendation 6 will improve the management of disability and the delivery of rehabilitation services to a large underserved portion of the US population. To achieve this objective will require modifying and expanding current education, training, and research programs in physical medicine and rehabilitation and rehabilitation science. The potential benefits are huge and will lead physicians in exciting new directions. Abraham Lincoln, a leader familiar with facing a long-standing challenge, suggested that the best way to predict the future is to create it.[39] Big data and the emerging field of data science provide the opportunity to create a better future for physical medicine and rehabilitation.

REFERENCES

1. Devy J. Online library. Sir Francis Bacon. The advancement of learning 1605. Book I, v.8.Available at: http://oll.libertyfund.org/titles/bacon-the-advancement-of-learning. Accessed July 3, 2018.

2. Weil AR. Big data in health: a new era for research and patient care. Health Aff 2014;33(7):1110.

3. King G. Ensuring the data-rich future of the social sciences. Science 2011;331: 719–21.

4. NIH strategic plan for data science. Available at: https://datascience.nih.gov/strategicplan. Accessed July 20, 2018.

5. Loukides M. What is data science? Cambridge (MA): O'Reilly Press; 2012.

6. Margolis R, Derr L, Dunn M, et al. The National Institutes of Health's Big Data to Knowledge (BD2K) initiative: capitalizing on biomedical big data. J Am Med Inform Assoc 2014;21(6):957–8.

7. Segal JB, Kapoor W, Carey T, et al. Preliminary competencies for comparative effectiveness research. Clin Transl Sci 2012;5(6):476–9.

8. NIH common fund: big data to knowledge (BD2K). Phase 1 and phase 2. Available at: https://commonfund.nih.gov/bd2k. Accessed June 15, 2018.

9. Jagodnik KM, Koplev S, Jenkins S, et al. Developing a framework for digital objects in the big data to knowledge (BD2K) commons: report from the commons framework pilots workshop. J Biomed Inform 2017;71:49–57.

10. Roski J, Bo-Lin GW, Andrews TA. Creating value in health care through big data: opportunities and policy implications. Health Aff 2014;33(7):1115–22.

11. The Mobilize Center. National Center Of Simulation in Rehabilitation Research. Stanford University. Available at: http://mobilize.stanford.edu/Accessed June 22, 2018.

12. Ottenbacher KJ, Karmarkar A, Graham JE. Thirty-day hospital readmission following discharge from postacute rehabilitation in fee-for-service Medicare patients. JAMA 2014;311(6):604–14.

13. Kim J, Yoon S, Kang JJ, et al. Research designs and statistical methods trends in the Annals of Rehabilitation Medicine. Ann Rehabil Med 2017;41(3):475–82.

14. 111th Congress. Patient Protection and Affordable Care Act PL 111-148. Washington, DC: U.S. Government Printing Office; 2010.

15. Burwell SM. Setting value-based payment goals: HHS efforts to improve U.S. health care. N Engl J Med 2015;372(10):897–9.

16. Improving Medicare post-acute care transformation act of 2014, PL 113-185. Available at: https://www.govtrack.us/congress/bills/113/hr4994. Accessed July 4, 2018.

17. DeJong G. Coming to terms with the IMPACT Act of 2014. Am J Occup Ther 2016;70(3). 7003090010p1–7003090010p6.

18. Tsai TC, Jha AK. Hospital consolidation, competition, and quality: is bigger necessarily better? JAMA 2014;312(1):29–30.

19. Hazra R, Tenney S, Shlionskaya A, et al. DASH, the data and specimen hub of the National Institute of Child Health and Human Development. Sci Data 2018;5: 180046.

20. PCORnet: national patient-centered clinical research network. Available at: http://www.pcornet.org/. Accessed June 22, 2018.

21. National Institutes of Health. The All Of Us Research Program. U.S. Department of Health and Human Services. Available at: https://allofus.nih.gov/. Accessed June 15, 2018.

22. Increasing access to the results of federally funded scientific research. Washington, DC: The White House Office of Science, Technology and Policy; U.S. Government; 2013. Available at: https://www.whitehouse.gov/blog/2013/02/22/expanding-public-access-results-federally-funded-research. Accessed June 2, 2018.

23. Institute of Medicine. Sharing clinical trial data: maximizing benefits, minimizing risk. Washington, DC: The National Academies Press; 2015.

24. Ross JS, Krumholz HM. Ushering in a new era of open science through data sharing: the wall must come down. JAMA 2013;309(13):1355–6.

25. Babbage D. Open and abundant data is the future of physical medicine and rehabilitation. Arch Phys Med Rehabil 2014;95:795–8.

26. Neylon C. Building a culture of data sharing: policy design and implementation for research data management in development research. Research Ideas and Outcomes 2017;3:e21773.

27. NIH Office of Extramural Research. NIH data sharing policy 2007. Available at: http://grants2.nih.gov/grants/policy/data_sharing/. Accessed March 15, 2018.

28. Agency for Healthcare Research and Quality. AHRQ public access to federally funded research 2015. Available at: http://www.ahrq.gov/funding/policies/publicaccess/index.html. Accessed May 25, 2017.

29. National Science Foundation. Office of Budget Finance & Award Management. Dissemination and Sharing of Research Results. Available at: https://www.nsf.gov/bfa/dias/policy/dmp.jsp. Accessed May 30, 2018.

30. AHRQ public access to federally funded research: publication and data. Rockville (MD): Agency for Healthcare Research and Quality; 2015. Available at: http://www.ahrq.gov/funding/policies/publicaccess/.

31. Federal Interagency Traumatic Brain Injury Research (FITBIR) informatics system. Available at: https://fitbir.nih.gov/. Accessed May 23, 2018.

32. Wilkinson MD, Dumontier M, Aalbersberg IJ, et al. The FAIR Guiding Principles for scientific data management and stewardship. Sci Data 2016;3:160018.

33. Biomedical and healthCAre Data Discovery Index Ecosystem (bioCADDIE). Supported by the National Institutes of Health, Big Data to Knowledge, Grant 1U24AI117966-01. Available at: https://datamed.org/index.php. Accessed August 9, 2018.

34. Center for Large Data Research and Data Sharing in Rehabilitation. University of Texas Medical Branch. Available at: https://www.utmb.edu/cldr Accessed June 21, 2018.

35. MR3 Medical Rehabilitation Research Resource Network. National Institutes of Health. Available at: https://ncmrr.org/. Accessed May 3, 2018.

36. Pope AM, Tralov AR. Disability in America: toward a national agenda for prevention. Washington, DC: National Academies Press; 1991.

37. Brandt EM, Pope A. Enabling America: assessing the role of rehabilitation science and engineering. Washington, DC: National Academy Press; 1997.

38. Field MJ, Jette AM. The future of disability in America. Washington, DC: National Academies Press; 2007.

39. Leidner GE. Abraham Lincoln: quotes, quips and speeches. Nashville (TN): Cumberland House; 2000.

Telemedicine in Rehabilitation

Marinella DeFre Galea, MD

KEYWORDS

- Telerehabilitation • Telehealth • Telemedicine

KEY POINTS

- Telemedicine offers the opportunity to deliver rehabilitative services in the patients' home, closing geographic, physical, and motivational gaps.
- The exponential growth of telerehabilitation has yielded the proliferation of studies with varying methodologies.
- Several methods of telerehabilitation delivery alone and in conjunction with traditional rehabilitation methodology have been explored based on available technology, patient literacy and level of function, and caregiver availability.

INTRODUCTION

In the past decade, the use of technology for remote assessment and intervention in rehabilitation has grown exponentially, paving the way for the development of telerehabilitation. The services provided under this term are wide in scope and can include evaluation, assessment, monitoring, prevention, intervention, supervision, education, consultation, and coaching. There is no formal structure for the delivery of telehealth, and the exchange of data may occur in numerous forms. Telephone, messaging and e-mail, or multimodal systems, such as videoconferencing, virtual therapists, and interactive Web-based platforms are some examples. In the field of rehabilitation, the patient-centered team approach has guided the identification of ad hoc solutions to overcome geographic, temporal, social, and financial barriers.[1]

Telerehabilitation has been shown to strengthen the patient-provider connection by (1) enhancing the knowledge of the patients and their contextual factors, (2) providing information exchange and facilitating education, and (3) establishing shared goal setting and action planning.[2] In the inpatient setting, telerehabilitation has been used to shorten hospital stay, facilitate discharge home, and provide patient and caregiver education and support.[3–5] In the outpatient setting, telemedicine supplements or

The author has nothing to disclose.

Department of Spinal Cord Injury and Disorder, Amyotrophic Lateral Sclerosis Program, Multiple Sclerosis Regional Center, The James J Peters VAMC, SCI/D Unit, 130 West Kingsbridge Road, Bronx, NY 10468, USA

E-mail address: Marinella.galea@va.gov

substitutes face-to-face encounters in acute and chronic neurologic, cardiac, and musculoskeletal conditions commonly treated by physiatrists.

As the application of telehealth proliferates, a central concern is how to protect data to preserve patient privacy. The Office of the National Coordination for Health Information Technology reported that health information is at a high risk for breaches, with more than 113 million individuals affected in 2015.[6] Although health care providers routinely receive mandatory training about how to safeguard the privacy and security of health care information during face-to-face encounters, the same is not true for virtual visits. In fact, very few studies have reported on the privacy and security of health care information in the context of telehealth. A systematic review by Peterson and colleague[7] shows that health care providers do not have a clear idea of how to protect health information when using telehealth. The investigators conclude that existing best practices are inconsistent across telehealth services and tools to assist health care providers are needed. To address this gap, the American Telemedicine Association (ATA) has recently developed a document to inform and assist practitioners in providing effective and secure telerehabilitation services, laying the foundation for developing discipline-specific standards, guidelines, and practice requirements.[8]

The development of a user-friendly, cost-effective, integrated telerehabilitation system aligned with existing policies will necessitate a business model that ensures effective, sustainable, and value-based services.[9] A forecast by Goldman Sachs estimates the comprehensive value of the US telerehabilitation market at $32.4 billion, of which 45% derives from remote patient monitoring; 37% from telehealth; and 18% from behavioral modifications.[10] Data from the QYR Pharma & Healthcare Research Center confirm the growth trend of the telerehabilitation market in the United States.[11] Cost-effectiveness has been shown in the application of tele-stroke,[12] cardiac rehabilitation,[13,14] traumatic brain injury,[15] and hip replacement rehabilitation.[4] Although insurance coverage for telerehabilitation services varies, the cost of technology is decreasing, making telerehabilitation modalities more affordable.[9] The 2017 ATA State Telemedicine Gap analysis[16] shows that, of the 37 states analyzed, 13 states do not cover telerehabilitation services for their Medicaid recipients. Although state policies vary in scope and application, 24 states reimburse for telerehabilitative services in their Medicaid plans. Only 12 states reimburse for telerehabilitative services within home health benefits.

This article presents recent applications of this burgeoning field of telerehabilitation by various medical subspecialties. These case studies demonstrate the evidence base for telerehabilitation, highlight potential areas of improvement, and propose potential future directions and applications.

CONTENT
Neurologic Telerehabilitation

The use of telemedicine in acute stroke has validated the proof-of-concept that specialized services can be delivered virtually when they cannot be easily provided face-to-face.[17] Several teleneurology applications have been proposed to manage patients with chronic neurologic diseases where impaired mobility hinders access.[18]

Stroke

Research has shown that more time spent on exercise therapy in the first weeks to months after stroke leads to better functioning.[19] Under the present health care system, transitional care programs are insufficient to address the barriers preventing community stroke survivors from achieving their highest potential, leading to hospital readmission, poorer outcome, and permanent disability.[20] Several randomized controlled trials have used alternative solutions to provide and/or supplement care in the patient's home after discharge.

Caregiver-delivered rehabilitation services have been evaluated to augment intensity of practice. A Cochrane review[21] showed that caregiver-mediated exercises (CME) administered alone or in combination with standard therapy have no significant effect on basic activities of daily living. However, CME significantly improved patients' standing balance and quality of life with no significant effects on caregiver strain. A more recent review showed that telerehabilitation interventions were associated with significant improvements in recovery from motor deficits, higher cortical dysfunction, and depression in the intervention groups in all studies assessed. Modalities used included tele-supervision, virtual reality, game-based virtual reality, and interactive mobile phone applications.[12]

Ongoing studies promise to provide more definitive evidence on CME and to assess the utility of televisits by the interdisciplinary team using more rigorous methodology.[22,23]

Approximately one-third of all people with stroke suffer from depressive symptoms,[24] using more health care services and increasing costs. In addition, the presence of depression is associated with poor functional outcomes after stroke.[24] Telerehabilitation has been successfully applied to address motor and nonmotor domains measured by the Stroke Impact Scale in a study comparing the effects of home-based robot-assisted rehabilitation coupled with a home exercise program versus home-based exercise alone.[25] The investigators were not able to determine why the quality-of-life and depression outcomes improved. They hypothesized that the positive trend could be attributed to the intervention per se, the resulting modest motor improvement, or the weekly interaction between the participants and the therapists.

Spinal cord injury

Individuals with spinal cord injury (SCI) experience substantial physical, psychological, and social challenges, requiring frequent, specialized, and interdisciplinary care. Several telerehabilitation modalities have been proposed to deliver specialized care and provide education and training. As described in a recent literature review,[26] to date there are a limited number of randomized controlled studies with different patient selection, outcomes, and modalities. The investigators conclude that there is not enough evidence about optimal methods of utilization, policy, and efficacy of telerehabilitation in SCI. Of note is that the reviewed studies showed high patient satisfaction and engagement.

Within the SCI system of care, the Veterans Health Administration (VHA) has developed a robust telehealth structure to address the postacute and chronic consequences of SCI. The Disease Management Protocol consist of semicustomized questions delivered to the patients' home via data messaging devices to evaluate changes in comorbidity severity and health-related quality of life.[27] The system has been shown to be most beneficial to newly injured patients recently discharged from acute rehabilitation that live far from specialty SCI care facilities. In recent years, the VHA has supported the use of Clinical Video Telehealth, a real-time videoconferencing system, to provide health care services. Qualitative analysis has shown that the system is complex and requires coordination and communication among stakeholders.[27,28] Video connect is a new secure provider to patient solution that is used to supplement face-to-face visits; data regarding its efficacy in delivering care and comparability with face-to-face encounters are not yet available. Notably, the VHA has invested in extensive health care provider education and training, constructed a safe and secure telemedicine structure, and marketed to its consumers.

Limited tele-exercise studies have been successfully executed in small cohorts of individuals with SCI.

One pilot study[29] used a platform consisting of a home monitoring system to record physiologic parameters, a hand ergometer to perform a customized home exercise program (HEP), and a tablet to conduct video training. The therapy sessions were led by a telecoach. Results showed 100% adherence to the HEP, that all participants experienced a modest improvement in aerobic capacity (24%), and physical activity and increased satisfaction with life scores. Subjects valued the motivation and disability-related expertise provided by the telecoach, consistent with the theory of Supportive Accountability,[30] which accounts for the complex interaction of a health care professional and consumer when communicating through electronic health technology.

Van Straaten and colleagues[31] studied the effectiveness of a HEP on pain and function. Results showed that after a 12-week intervention consisting of a high-dose scapular stabilizer and rotator cuff strengthening program using telerehabilitation for supervision, shoulder pain was reduced even in individuals with longstanding symptoms. The study was limited by sample size, lack of a control group, and low to moderate levels of pain at baseline.

Video visits have been used in SCI to provide nonurgent specialized consultation in lieu of, or in addition to, face-to-face visits. A recent pilot study[32] using iPads in the SCI population confirmed previous findings[33,34] that videoconferencing is a clinically viable and effective tool. The type of interactions between clinicians and participants varied from generalized hospital follow-up and SCI–primary care to specific questions on medications and coordination with subspecialty clinics. This modality has been well-accepted by patients and caregivers and has reduced rate of hospitalization and overall length of stay.

Multiple sclerosis

Individuals with multiple sclerosis (MS) are at risk for developing long-term disability. Rehabilitation provides treatments and therapies to lessen the impact of disability and improve function; however, access to those services is complicated by limited mobility, fatigue, and related issues. It has been shown that individuals with MS are willing to receive rehabilitative services through telemedicine. However, patients with moderate-to-severe disability may experience technical difficulties due to cognitive and physical impairment.[35]

Charvet and colleagues[36] have used an adaptive online cognitive improvement program to train individuals with MS at home. The patients were randomly assigned to either a conventional adaptive cognitive remediation program or an active control of ordinary computer games. This telerehabilitation modality provided modest improvement in cognitive performance as measured by changes in a composite of neuropsychological tests.

Khan and colleagues[37] conducted a systematic review of the use of telerehabilitation to provide or supplement therapy to individuals with MS. The studies evaluated included multiple delivery modalities, some complex, with more than one rehabilitation component and included physical activity, educational, behavioral, and symptom management programs. With such heterogeneous methodology, it was concluded that there is limited evidence on the efficacy of telerehabilitation in improving functional activities, fatigue, and quality of life in adults with MS. The review also found that evidence supporting telerehabilitation in the longer term for improved function, impairment, quality of life, and psychological outcomes is poor. A very recent randomized trial[38] provides higher-quality evidence that telerehabilitation is technically feasible, desirable, and effective in improving gait and other outcomes in patients with MS.

An ongoing study is evaluating the delivery of complementary and alternative medicine sessions at home to rural and low-income individuals with MS versus the same intervention delivered in the clinic by a therapist.[39]

Traumatic brain injury

It has been shown that many people with traumatic brain injury (TBI) are interested in accessing telerehabilitative services to assist with problems in memory, attention, problem-solving, and activities of daily living.[40] In addition, as their caregivers assume increased responsibility for providing support, they receive limited access to services leading to increased risk of anxiety and depression.[41]

Rietdijk and colleagues[42] conducted a systematic review searching for interventions delivered at distance with the use of technology, involving caregivers of adults and children with TBI. They concluded that telehealth can be used to increase access to services for families in rural areas, to train family members in the skills required to facilitate recovery after TBI, to provide appropriate and timely intervention for problems arising at home, or to create a forum for peer support. Significant outcomes included improved cognitive functioning of the person with TBI as well as psychological well-being, support skills, and burden of caregivers. Several studies demonstrated that participants reported training to be beneficial over the long-term after program completion, and that improvements in outcomes were maintained over time.

A more recent systematic review by Ownsworth and colleagues[15] aimed to determine whether telerehabilitation interventions are effective for improving outcomes relative to usual care, alternative interventions, and baseline functioning. Of the modalities described, telephone interventions focused on managing self-identified concerns through tailored interventions, providing education and strategies for enhancing cognitive skills and physical exercise, and encouraging compliance with prescribed therapy, were most used. Of interest, Web-based platforms were rarely used compared with other neurologic conditions, possibly because of TBI-related impairments and dependence on caregiver assistance. Telephone-based interventions were found to improve global functioning, posttraumatic symptoms, sleep quality, and depressive symptoms for individuals with mild and moderate-to-severe TBI relative to usual care; however, the durability of these effects was either not demonstrated or not examined by these studies.

Cardiac Telerehabilitation

Coronary artery disease

Cardiac rehabilitation has beneficial effects on morbidity and mortality in patients with coronary artery disease (CAD); however, it is underused and short-term improvements are often not sustained. Several randomized controlled trials[13,14] have shown that telerehabilitation provided positive results when compared with conventional hospital rehabilitation. Of interest, these studies use a combination of communication technologies (Internet, video-consultation), on-demand coaching to encourage compliance, and individually tailored coaching on both training intensity and physical activity.[43] Frederix and colleagues[14] have shown that a prolonged (1 year), Internet-based comprehensive telerehabilitation program in addition to conventional cardiac rehabilitation is cost-effective, and can reduce cardiovascular rehospitalization.

Congestive heart failure

In a recent study by Hwang and colleagues,[44] patients with stable congestive heart failure were randomized to 12 weeks of real-time exercise and education intervention using online videoconferencing software versus a traditional hospital-outpatient program. The group-based video telerehabilitation program was noninferior to an outpatient rehabilitation program and promoted greater attendance yielding few adverse effects. These findings confirm previous reports[45,46] that telerehabilitation is a safe care delivery modality. Similarly, Nouryan and colleagues[47] conducted a randomized controlled trial, studying Medicare outpatients with heart failure after discharge from home care for 6 months. Patients were randomized to home telehealth or comprehensive outpatient management. The telehealth intervention consisted of weekly televisits and daily vital signs monitoring. The results showed that the telehealth intervention group improved all causes of emergency department utilization, length of stay, and quality of life. A trend toward cost savings was reported in the telehealth intervention group; however, it did not reach statistical significance.

Musculoskeletal

Orthopedic care provides a fertile ground for the utilization of telerehabilitation in an aging population prone to osteoarthritis. In fact, procedures involving the musculoskeletal system are among the most common in the United States.[48] These interventions are paired with a rehabilitation program aimed at maximizing functional outcome.

A recent systematic review[49] identified several studies in which postsurgical telerehabilitation programs were implemented after total knee arthroplasty,[50] total hip arthroplasty,[4] and upper limb and hand surgeries.[51] Methods of administration included real-time videoconferencing, asynchronous programs, telephone follow-up, and interactive virtual systems. The investigators found strong evidence in favor of telerehabilitation in patients following total knee and hip arthroplasty and limited evidence in the upper limb interventions. Another review by Cottrell and colleagues[52] analyzed evidence exclusively for the use of real-time telerehabilitation for the treatment of musculoskeletal conditions. The investigators concluded that there was strong evidence that the management of musculoskeletal conditions via real-time telerehabilitation is effective in improving physical function, disability, and pain. At least one study has been proposed to study the delivery of a pre-habilitation program in surgical candidates awaiting total hip or knee arthroplasty, to address the reported long wait times before surgery.[53] Results are pending.

Occupational therapists often assess a patient's home for safety before discharge as part of their role in acute care and rehabilitation teams.[54] When the evaluation cannot be completed in a timely manner, delays in discharge and increased length of stay ensue, or the patient is discharged without the assessment, potentially leading to an increased risk of early readmission. The World Federation of Occupational Therapists has published a position statement on the use of telehealth to improve accessibility to occupational therapy. Telehealth has been suggested as an effective and reliable way to access home modification services.[55] Nix and Comans[5] described an initiative to improve the timeliness of occupational therapy home visits for discharge planning by implementing technology solutions while maintaining patient safety. The project demonstrated that on-site home visits can be safely and efficiently performed or augmented using technology. The study also highlighted the positive impact of the project on the occupational therapy department productivity.

Chronic Pain

Chronic pain is a major public health problem, which is expected to increase as the population ages. Physical training has been proven to decrease pain and improve function[56] and therefore plays an important role in current pain rehabilitation programs. Improvements in chronic low back pain seen in physical therapy do not appear to be retained over the long term, providing an opportunity for telerehabilitation services to provide continuity and ensure sustainability.[57]

Patients with chronic pain were favorable to an "intermediate" telerehabilitation program offering feedback and monitoring technology with some face-to-face consulting and exercise location.[58] However, Adamse and colleagues[59] conducted a systematic review of exercise-based telemedicine in patients with chronic pain and found no difference compared with usual care on physical activity, activities of daily living, and quality of life.

Telerehabilitation interventions have proven to be beneficial to retain improvement in low back pain and increase attrition, respectively, via booster sessions delivered through a mobile phone application[57] and videoconferencing.[60]

For patients with chronic knee pain, an Internet-delivered, physiotherapist-prescribed home exercise and pain-coping skills training provided clinically meaningful and sustained improvements in pain and function.[61]

Virtual complementary and integrative health modalities, such as yoga and tai chi sessions, to treat chronic pain are being investigated.

Rheumatology

A recent systematic review[62] shows that telemedicine has been applied to the field of rheumatology in the form of remote consultations, monitoring of treatment strategies, and Web-based self-management programs. Some of the chronic conditions treated include rheumatoid arthritis, systemic sclerosis, fibromyalgia, osteoarthritis, and juvenile idiopathic arthritis. Types of intervention have included remote disease activity assessment, tele-monitoring of treatment strategies, and information communication technology–delivered self-management programs.

In the application of tele-consultation, it was concluded that this modality resulted in high patient satisfaction rates, albeit lacking in diagnostic accuracy. Internet-delivered programs revealed high feasibility and satisfaction rates, although effectiveness data lacked homogeneity. Remote monitoring programs were also well received by patients. Cost-effectiveness needs to be evaluated, as readmission rates were higher in patients on tight control and treat-to-target approaches. Self-directed kinesiotherapy sessions were effective in improving hand function after drug-induced remission.

In a recent study by Pani and colleagues,[63] the patients reported increased motivation and greater engagement of the medical staff in their therapy when using an ad hoc telerehabilitation platform. Although the investigators did not perform a formal cost analysis, they concluded that the proposed solution appeared to be cost-effective compared with face-to-face therapy sessions.

SUMMARY

Studies have provided evidence that telerehabilitation is well received by patients whether applied alone or to supplement conventional therapy; it does not add burden to the caregiver; it is advantageous for patients recovering from motor deficits, higher cortical dysfunction, and depression after stroke; and to recover after hip and knee arthroplasty.

Lack of methodological rigor and variability of approaches used in telerehabilitation studies to date hinder the ability to conclude that telehealth services can and should be deployed more broadly in the delivery of rehabilitation.

Larger, well-powered, longer-term studies are needed to provide definitive evidence and establish the indications and limitations of telerehabilitation utilization in the treatment of acute and chronic conditions.

There is a need for best practices that are consistent across all types of telehealth services for all health care providers. In this rapidly evolving field, existing research may not reflect the most recent developments in practice or technology and best practice may be moving ahead of the research reported in publications.

Strong, evidence-based telerehabilitation methodologies together with best practices will provide the matrix to create effective services that can be both delivered by health care structures and reimbursed by health insurance providers.

REFERENCES

1. Hailey D, Roine R, Ohinmaa A, et al. Evidence of benefit from telerehabilitation in routine care: a systematic review. J Telemed Telecare 2011;17(6):281–7.
2. Wang S, Blazer D, Hoenig H. Can eHealth technology enhance the patient-provider relationship in rehabilitation? Arch Phys Med Rehabil 2016;97(9): 1403–6.
3. Tsavourelou A, Stylianides N, Papadopoulos A, et al. Telerehabilitation solution conceptual paper for community-based exercise rehabilitation of patients discharged after critical illness. Int J Telerehabil 2016;8(2):61–70.
4. Nelson M, Bourke M, Crossley K, et al. Telerehabilitation versus traditional care following total hip replacement: a randomized controlled trial protocol. JMIR Res Protoc 2017;6(3):e34.
5. Nix J, Comans T. Home quick–occupational therapy home visits using mHealth, to facilitate discharge from acute admission back to the community. Int J Telerehabil 2017;9(1):47–54.
6. Office of the National Coordinator for Health Information Technology. Breaches of unsecured protected health information. Health IT Quick-Stat #53. 2016. Available at: https://dashboard.healthit.gov/quickstats/pages/breaches-protected-health-informatio.
7. Peterson C, Watzlaf V. Telerehabilitation store and forward applications: a review of applications and privacy considerations in physical and occupational therapy practice. Int J Telerehabil 2015;6(2):75–84.
8. Richmond T, Peterson C, Cason J, et al. American Telemedicine Association's principles for delivering telerehabilitation services. Int J Telerehabil 2017;9(2): 63–8.
9. Marzano G, Ochoa-Siguencia L, Pellegrino A. Towards a new wave of telerehabilitation applications. The Open Public Health Journal 2017;1(1):1–9.
10. The digital revolution comes to US Healthcare. 2015. Available at: www.Wur.Nl/Upload_mm/0/f/3/8fe8684c-2a84-4965-9dce-550584aae48c_Internet%20of%20Things%205%20-%20Digital%20Revolution%20Comes%20to%20US%20Healtcare.Pdf.
11. QYR Pharma & Healthcare Research Center. Global and United States telerehabilitation systems market size, status and forecast 2022. 2017.
12. Sarfo FS, Ulasavets U, Opare-Sem OK, et al. Tele-rehabilitation after stroke: an updated systematic review of the literature. J Stroke Cerebrovasc Dis 2018; 27(9):2306–18.
13. Frederix I, Solmi F, Piepoli MF, et al. Cardiac telerehabilitation: a novel cost-efficient care delivery strategy that can induce long-term health benefits. Eur J Prev Cardiol 2017;24(16):1708–17.
14. Frederix I, Vandijck D, Hens N, et al. Economic and social impact of increased cardiac rehabilitation uptake and cardiac telerehabilitation in Belgium—a cost–benefit analysis. Acta Cardiolo 2017;73(3):222–9.

15. Ownsworth T, Arnautovska U, Beadle E, et al. Efficacy of telerehabilitation for adults with traumatic brain injury: a systematic review. J Head Trauma Rehabil 2017;33(4):E33–46.
16. Capistrant G, Thomas L. State telemedicine gaps analysis: coverage and reimbursement. American Telehealth Association 2017. Available at: https://utn.org/resources/downloads/50-state-telemedicine-gaps-analysis-physician-practice-standards-licensure.pdf.
17. Schwamm LH, Pancioli A, Acker JE, et al. American Stroke Association's Task force on the development of stroke systems. Recommendations for the establishment of stroke systems of care: recommendations from the American Stroke Association's task force on the development of stroke systems. Circulation 2005; 111(8):1078–91.
18. Wechsler LR, Tsao JW, Levine SR, et al, American Academy of Neurology Telemedicine Work Group. Teleneurology applications: report of the telemedicine work group of the American Academy of Neurology. Neurology 2013;80(7):670–6.
19. English C, Veerbeek J. Is more physiotherapy better after stroke? Int J Stroke 2015;10(4):465–6.
20. Lichtman JH, Leifheit-Limson EC, Jones SB, et al. Preventable readmissions within 30 days of ischemic stroke among Medicare beneficiaries. Stroke 2013; 44(12):3429–35.
21. Vloothuis JDM, Mulder M, Veerbeek JM, et al. Caregiver-mediated exercises for improving outcomes after stroke. Cochrane Database Syst Rev 2016;(12):CD011058.
22. Vloothius J, Mulder M, Nijland RH. Caregiver-mediated exercises with e-health support for early supported discharge after stroke (CARE4STROKE): study protocol for a randomized controlled trial. BMC Neurol 2017;15:193.
23. Jhaveri MM, Benjamin-Garner R, Rianon N, et al. Telemedicine-guided education on secondary stroke and fall prevention following inpatient rehabilitation for Texas patients with stroke and their caregivers: a feasibility pilot study. BMJ Open 2017; 7(9):e017340.
24. Wulsin L, Alwell K, Moomaw CJ, et al. Comparison of two depression measures for predicting stroke outcomes. J Psychosom Res 2012;72(3):175–9.
25. Linder SM, Rosenfeldt AB, Bay RC, et al. Improving quality of life and depression after stroke through telerehabilitation. Am J Occup Ther 2015;69(2). 6902290020p1-10.
26. Irgens I, Rekand T, Arora M, et al. Telehealth for people with spinal cord injury: a narrative review. Spinal Cord 2018;56(7):643–55.
27. Woo C, Seton JM, Washington M, et al. Increasing specialty care access through use of an innovative home telehealth-based spinal cord injury disease management protocol (SCI DMP). J Spinal Cord Med 2016;39(1):3–12.
28. Martinez RN, Hogan TP, Balbale S, et al. Sociotechnical perspective on implementing clinical video telehealth for veterans with spinal cord injuries and disorders. Telemed J E Health 2017;23(7):567–76.
29. Lai B, Rimmer J, Barstow B, et al. Teleexercise for persons with spinal cord injury: a mixed-methods feasibility case series. JMIR Rehabil Assist Technol 2016;3(2):e8.
30. Mohr DC, Cuijpers P, Lehman K. Supportive accountability: a model for providing human support to enhance adherence to eHealth interventions. J Med Internet Res 2011;13(1):e30.
31. Van Straaten MG, Cloud BA, Morrow MM, et al. Effectiveness of home exercise on pain, function, and strength of manual wheelchair users with spinal cord injury: a high-dose shoulder program with telerehabilitation. Arch Phys Med Rehabil 2014; 95(10):1810–7.e2.

32. Shem K, Sechrist SJ, Loomis E, et al. SCiPad: effective implementation of tele-medicine using iPads with individuals with spinal cord injuries, a case series. Front Med (Lausanne) 2017;4:58.

33. Veerbeek JM, Van Wegen E, Van Peppen R, et al. What is the evidence for phys-ical therapy poststroke? A systematic review and meta-analysis. PLoS One 2014; 9(2):e87987.

34. Phillips VL, Vesmarovich S, Hauber R, et al. Telehealth: reaching out to newly injured spinal cord patients. Public Health Rep 2001;116(Suppl 1):94–102.

35. Remy C, Valet M, Stoquart G. Telecommunication and rehabilitation among pa-tients with multiple sclerosis: access and willingness to use. Ann Phys Rehabil Med 2018;61:e99.

36. Charvet LE, Yang J, Shaw MT, et al. Cognitive function in multiple sclerosis im-proves with telerehabilitation: results from a randomized controlled trial. PLoS One 2017;12(5):e0177177.

37. Khan F, Amatya B, Kesselring J, et al. Telerehabilitation for persons with multiple sclerosis. Cochrane Database Syst Rev 2015;(4):CD010508.

38. Conroy SS, Zhan M, Culpepper WJ, et al. Self directed exercise in multiple scle-rosis: Evaluation of a home automated tele-management system. J Telemed Tele-care 2018;24(6):410–9.

39. Rimmer J, Thirumalai M, Young H, et al. Rationale and design of the tele-exercise and multiple sclerosis (TEAMS) study: a comparative effectiveness trial between a clinic- and home-based telerehabilitation intervention for adults with multiple scle-rosis (MS) living in the deep south. Contemp Clin Trials Commun 2018;71:186–93.

40. Ricker JH, Rosenthal M, Garay E, et al. Telerehabilitation needs: a survey of per-sons with acquired brain injury. J Head Trauma Rehabil 2002;17(3):242–50.

41. Kreutzer JS, Rapport LJ, Marwitz JH, et al. Caregivers' well-being after traumatic brain injury: a multicenter prospective investigation. Arch Phys Med Rehabil 2009;90(6):939–46.

42. Rietdijk R, Togher L, Power E. Supporting family members of people with trau-matic brain injury using telehealth: A systematic review. Journal of Rehabilitation Medicine 2012;44:913–21.

43. Brouwers RWM, Kraal JJ, Traa SCJ, et al. Effects of cardiac telerehabilitation in patients with coronary artery disease using a personalised patient-centred web application: protocol for the SmartCare-CAD randomised controlled trial. BMC Cardiovasc Disord 2017;17(1):46.

44. Hwang R, Bruning J, Morris NR, et al. Home-based telerehabilitation is not inferior to a centre-based program in patients with chronic heart failure: a randomised trial. J Physiother 2017;63(2):101–7.

45. Piotrowicz E, Baranowski R, Bilinska M, et al. A new model of home-based tele-monitored cardiac rehabilitation in patients with heart failure: effectiveness, qual-ity of life, and adherence. Eur J Heart Fail 2010;12(2):164–71.

46. Piotrowicz E, Zieliłski T, Bodalski R, et al. Home-based telemonitored Nordic walking training is well accepted, safe, effective and has high adherence among heart failure patients, including those with cardiovascular implantable electronic devices: a randomised controlled study. Eur J Prev Cardiol 2015;22(11):1368–77.

47. Nouryan C, Morahan S, Pecinka K, et al. Home telemonitoring of community-dwelling heart failure patients after home care discharge. Telemed J E Health 2018. [Epub ahead of print].

48. Fingar KR, Stocks C, Weiss AJ, et al. Most frequent operating room procedures performed in U.S. Hospitals, 2003–2012. HCUP statistical brief #186. Rockville (MD): Agency for Healthcare Research and Quality; 2014.

49. Kairy D, Lehoux P, Vincent C, et al. A systematic review of clinical outcomes, clinical process, healthcare utilization and costs associated with telerehabilitation. Disabil Rehabil 2009;31(6):427–47.
50. Moffet H, Tousignant M, Nadeau S, et al. Patient satisfaction with in-home telerehabilitation after total knee arthroplasty: results from a randomized controlled trial. Telemed J E Health 2017;23(2):80–7.
51. Pastora-Bernal JM, Martín-Valero R, Barón-López FJ, et al. Evidence of benefit of telerehabilitation after orthopedic surgery: a systematic review. J Med Internet Res 2017;19(4):e142.
52. Cottrell MA, Galea OA, O'Leary SP, et al. Real-time telerehabilitation for the treatment of musculoskeletal conditions is effective and comparable to standard practice: a systematic review and meta-analysis. Clin Rehabil 2017;31(5):625–38.
53. Doiron-Cadrin P, Kairy D, Vendittoli PA, et al. Effects of a tele-prehabilitation program or an in-person prehabilitation program in surgical candidates awaiting total hip or knee arthroplasty: protocol of a pilot single blind randomized controlled trial. Contemp Clin Trials Commun 2016;4:192–8.
54. Cumming RG, Thomas M, Szonyi G, et al. Home visits by an occupational therapist for assessment and modification of environmental hazards: a randomized trial of falls prevention. J Am Geriatr Soc 1999;47(12):1397–402.
55. World Federation of Occupational Therapists. World Federation of Occupational Therapists' position statement on telehealth. Int J Telerehabil 2014;6(1):37–9.
56. Van Tulder M, Malmivaara A, Esmail R, et al. Exercise therapy for low back pain: a systematic review within the framework of the Cochrane collaboration back review group. Spine (Phila Pa 1976) 2000;25(21):2784–96.
57. Peterson S. Telerehabilitation booster sessions and remote patient monitoring in the management of chronic low back pain: a case series. Physiother Theory Pract 2018;34(5):393–402.
58. Cranen K, Groothuis-Oudshoorn CGM, Vollenbroek-Hutten MMR, et al. Toward patient-centered telerehabilitation design: understanding chronic pain patients' preferences for web-based exercise telerehabilitation using a discrete choice experiment. J Med Internet Res 2017;19(1):e26.
59. Adamse C, Dekker-Van Weering MG, van Etten-Jamaludin FS, et al. The effectiveness of exercise-based telemedicine on pain, physical activity and quality of life in the treatment of chronic pain: a systematic review. J Telemed Telecare 2018; 24(8):511–26.
60. Herbert MS, Afari N, Liu L, et al. Telehealth versus in-person acceptance and commitment therapy for chronic pain: a randomized noninferiority trial. J Pain 2017;18(2):200–11.
61. Bennell KL, Nelligan R, Dobson F, et al. Effectiveness of an Internet-delivered exercise and pain-coping skills training intervention for persons with chronic knee pain: a randomized trial. Ann Intern Med 2017;166(7):453–62.
62. Piga M, Cangemi I, Mathieu A, et al. Telemedicine for patients with rheumatic diseases: systematic review and proposal for research agenda. Semin Arthritis Rheum 2017. https://doi.org/10.1016/j.semarthrit.2017.03.014.
63. Pani D, Piga M, Barabino G, et al. Home tele-rehabilitation for rheumatic patients: impact and satisfaction of care analysis. J Telemed Telecare 2017;23(2):292–300.

Apps and Mobile Health Technology in Rehabilitation
The Good, the Bad, and the Unknown

Lindsay Ramey, MD*, Candice Osborne, PhD, MPH, OTR, Donald Kasitinon, MD, Shannon Juengst, PhD, CRC

KEYWORDS

- Mobile health (mHealth) • Smartphone • Applications (apps) • Technology
- Rehabilitation

KEY POINTS

- Despite high smartphone ownership rates, there is disparity in current access to mHealth services among individuals with disabilities.
- Mobile health interventions have the potential to provide evidence-based education, promote self-management, support specific rehabilitation goals, and monitor biometrics and symptoms, although evidence to date is lacking.
- Many products are available that may benefit individuals with disabilities, although content, quality, and accessibility are variable, and less than 1% of commercially available mHealth apps are evidence-based.
- Literature supporting the clinical efficacy of mHealth interventions within rehabilitation medicine is most robust for cardiac rehabilitation, mental health disorders, and brain injury.
- Research in rehabilitation medicine is largely limited to small feasibility and pilot studies.

INTRODUCTION

According to the World Health Organization, mobile health (mHealth) technology is "medical and public health practice supported by mobile devices," including wearables, portable digital assistants (PDAs), handheld computers, smartphones, and tablets. This article focuses on application (app)-based mHealth technologies for smartphones and tablets. Although mHealth apps are often criticized for serving only those with mobile phone access and/or operator knowledge, smartphone

The authors have nothing to disclose.
Department of Physical Medicine and Rehabilitation, University of Texas Southwestern Medical Center in Dallas, 5161 Harry Hines Boulevard, Charles Sprague Building, CS6.104, Dallas, TX 75390, USA
* Corresponding author.
E-mail address: Lindsay.ramey@utsouthwestern.edu

technology is rapidly becoming ubiquitous. As of 2016, smartphones were owned by 92% of individuals in the United States ages 18 to 29, 88% of those ages 30 to 49, and 74% of those ages 50 to 64. Of those aged 65 and older, 42% had smartphones in 2016,[1] with that number increasing to 67% in 2017.[2] In 2016, 77% of all US adults owned a smartphone, dramatically up from 35% in 2011.[1] Smartphone devices are currently owned by 64% of those earning less than $30,000 per year and 54% of those with less than a high school education, with no differences in ownership among racial and ethnic groups.[1]

The use of mainstream wireless technologies in health management has grown exponentially in the last decade, with more than 325,000 mHealth apps available in 2017, up 25% since 2016.[3] Most mHealth apps focus on fitness (36%), stress management (17%), and diet (12%), with the remaining 35% focused on disease management.[4] Patients and health care providers are increasingly using mHealth apps to support health and wellness. Ninety-six percent of current mHealth users report that mHealth has improved their quality of life.[5] More than 50% of individuals not using mHealth services believe that such technologies would improve the quality and/or decrease the cost of their health care within the next 3 years, and 70% of physicians report that mHealth apps encourage patients to take more responsibility of their own health.[5,6]

MOBILE HEALTH DISPARITY AMONG PEOPLE WITH DISABILITIES

Discrepancies have been reported in smartphone ownership and mHealth use among people with disabilities (PWD). According to the Pew Research Center, 58% of Americans with disabilities own a smartphone and 36% own a tablet (compared with 77% and 54% of all adults, respectively).[7] In contrast, the 2016 Survey of User Needs reported higher ownership rates, similar to the general population, among PWDs: 70% and 50% for smartphone and tablet ownership, respectively.[8] However, within the general population, 34% of smartphone owners report that they have downloaded an app to track or manage health metrics, whereas among PWD, this rate drops to 17%.[6,9] There are likely multiple factors contributing to this discrepancy; two likely factors are presented next.

In a 2017 survey of 377 regular Internet users with a disability, more than half (54%) reported accessible apps were hard to find.[9] A recent study examined accessibility of iOS-based blood pressure or blood glucose monitoring apps and found none to be accessible based on Apple's current accessibility guidelines or Section 408 of the Rehabilitation Act.[10] A literature review from 2008 to 2017 sought to identify peer-reviewed assessments of mHealth apps for PWDs.[6] Despite reviewing 91 articles, only three mHealth apps were found that were evaluated by PWD (iMHere, mCare, and IIAM). The small number of products developed for, evaluated by, and accessible to this population highlights a gap in current mHealth development likely contributing to this disparity.

Lack of awareness and appropriate training in the use of mHealth apps by PWD, particularly those with cognitive or mobility impairments that may require special accommodations, may further propagate this disparity, as illustrated by two recent surveys. The first, including 29 patients with traumatic brain injury (TBI), reported that only 10% of participants had received any instruction by a clinician regarding use of a smartphone.[11] The second, among health care professionals working with children and adolescents with brain injury (BI), reported that although 75% of the patients used mHealth services, only 42% of providers discussed or facilitated use of mHealth services among their patients.[12]

CURRENT EVIDENCE-BASE OF MOBILE HEALTH AND SMARTPHONE APPLICATIONS

Mhealth has the potential to efficiently and cost-effectively reach a large number of individuals (including currently underserved populations), improve clinical outcomes, promote attendance and adherence for health-behavior interventions, and improve health-related quality of life.[13–17] However, there is a concerning lack of evidence to support the efficacy of most commercially available mHealth apps, especially with regard to effecting sustainable improvements. There are thousands of mHealth apps available for download, and less than 1% of them are grounded in research evidence.[17,18] As with many emerging technologies, the development of mHealth applications tends to be commercially, rather than scientifically, driven.[17,18] This has the advantages of a rapid turn-around time from development to download and a wide variety of choices to suit any individual preference, but may do nothing for effectively improving health and health management over time. Despite the proliferation of untested apps, enough of an evidence-base has accumulated to support several systematic reviews of mHealth use in mental health and chronic disease management.[13,15,17,19,20] All of these systematic reviews conclude that mHealth supports short-term health-management improvements, but there remains a need for more evidence, particularly on long-term effects and maintenance of these improvements.[13,15,17,19–21] Ultimately, mHealth apps, paired with traditional health care delivery, may improve intervention outcomes and health-related quality of life, but requires practitioners to make informed recommendations regarding use of mHealth apps.

Regardless of medical specialty, mHealth apps can offer multiple different functions to aid in medical care:

1. Provide evidence-based education
2. Support compliance with specific medical treatment plans (eg, medications, appointments, exercise)
3. Support self- and clinician-monitoring of biometrics (heart rate, blood pressure, activity) and progress
4. Facilitate patient-provider communication (one-way or two-way)
5. Promote comprehensive self-management

The literature to date reveals limited use of mHealth apps to deliver or support medical rehabilitation. Most literature on mHealth interventions in rehabilitation has used telephone-based interventions. Most studies with positive results have used telephone calls or video conferencing with two-way communication between patient and provider rather than making use of the remote technology available in smartphones.[22–32] Because most mHealth apps offer limited two-way communication between patient and provider, it is difficult to generalize the positive results of these prior studies to emerging mHealth apps.

As technology evolves, the research to understand its role in medical care must evolve. Although many domains of rehabilitation medicine have the potential to be impacted by mHealth technologies, additional engagement from qualified health care providers is needed for product development, research design, and content oversight to ensure accessible, evidence-based, effective products are available.

PATIENT-CENTERED MOBILE HEALTH APPLICATIONS IN REHABILITATION MEDICINE
Mobile Health for Comprehensive Self-Management

Development of mobile apps to support self-monitoring and maintenance of health and well-being is rapidly growing.[33] The Institute of Medicine describes self-management support as "the systematic provision of education and supportive interventions by health care staff to increase patients' skills and confidence in managing their health problems, including regular assessment of progress and problems, goal setting, and problem-solving support."[34] A total of 69% of US adults track at least one health indicator, and individuals diagnosed with a chronic condition are significantly more likely to track health indicators compared with those without a chronic condition.[35]

Most mHealth apps are narrowly focused to assist with management of one specific aspect of health (ie, weight loss, blood glucose management) using a single function.[33] Few mHealth apps comprehensively support self-management of a chronic condition, which includes medical management, maintenance of meaningful behaviors or life roles, and management of the emotional symptoms.[36]

One example of a comprehensive mHealth system is the Interactive Mobile Health and Rehabilitation, or iMHere, app (not yet available for public download), used to augment services provided by the rehabilitation health care team. It guides users to set goals in six areas (**Fig. 1**):

1. Medication management
2. Bowel management
3. Bladder management
4. Skin integrity
5. Mood
6. Nutrition

It offers multiple functions to support these goals, including calendars and notifications for specific self-care tasks, biometric and progress tracking, patient education, and two-way patient-provider communication.[37] In a recent randomized controlled trial (RCT), use of iMHere was associated with improvements in self-management skills.[37] iMHere serves as an exemplar to address the substantial gaps in the current literature, including limited knowledge of self-management app development and implementation processes, user-centered design, long-term

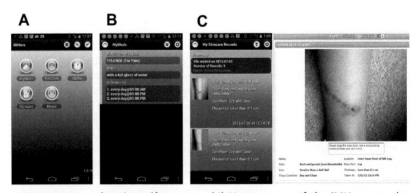

Fig. 1. iMHere comprehensive self-care app. (*A*) Home screen of the iMHere app demonstrating the multiple domains of care supported. (*B*) Medication domain of self-care with demonstration of the app providing information to the patient about medication frequency and instructions. (*C*) Skincare domain of self-care with demonstration of the app for data input by the patient on the *left* and demonstration of the clinical portal displaying data to the health care provider on the *right*. (*From* Parmanto B, Pramana G, Yu DX, et al. Originally published in JMIR mHealth and uHealth. 2013. Available at: http://mhealth.jmir.org. Accessed July 15, 2018; with permission.)

effectiveness, and organizational readiness to accept mHealth intervention in rehabilitation.[38]

Mobile Health for Weight Management

Obesity, inactivity, and poor nutrition are risk factors for many diagnoses encountered in rehabilitation medicine.[39] Many mHealth interventions are available to support weight management. A 2013 RCT of 70 adults in a weight management program showed that the addition of mHealth tracking (using a PDA) resulted in a 3.1% greater mean weight loss compared with standard care alone, with higher frequency of mHealth use leading to greater reductions in weight, body mass index, body fat percentage, and waist circumference.[40,41] A 2017 systematic review assessed the effectiveness of mHealth methods for improving obesity and diabetes self-management. Of the 24 studies included, eight focused on the use of an app (eg, *B*-MOBILE, SmartLossSM, MyFitnessPal).[42,43] Four of the eight studies reported significant improvement in outcomes with use of an app, although outcome measures varied. Interventions that targeted physical activity were most effective, followed by those that targeted diet. Short-term studies had more positive findings, and long-term interventions had higher drop-out rates raising the question of sustainable user engagement.[43]

Although the current evidence is promising, many mHealth weight management apps lack evidence of effectiveness, particularly long-term, and may contain misinformation.[44] The accessibility of weight management apps for PWD has not been studied; it remains unclear which apps are user-friendly for specific rehabilitation populations.

Mobile Health Interventions for Specific Diagnoses

Brain injury

mHealth apps present a unique, readily available, and potentially powerful tool to support individuals with BI, including acquired BI (ABI) and TBI. Evidence using older technologies (eg, PDA) suggests that mobile technology use is feasible and potentially effective for managing various long-term symptoms in chronic TBI.[11,45] However, technology development outpaces clinical research, and these older devices have become obsolete, replaced by smartphones as the primary platform for mHealth. Smartphones offer many advantages over older platforms in this population. They are portable, socially acceptable, and multifunctional, and given the ubiquitous use in today's society, most individuals are already familiar with the platform, which may improve ease of use, particularly in those with cognitive impairment. One pilot study of 17 adults with chronic TBI examined the feasibility of using a smartphone app for daily assessment of mood-related symptoms after TBI over 8 weeks. Daily compliance was 73.4%, and participants reported high satisfaction and ease of use.[46]

Most task-specific mHealth services for individuals with ABI target memory impairment. Two systematic reviews on mHealth use for individuals with memory impairment and ABI concluded that technology to support memory could improve performance on daily activities.[11,45] A recent review of mHealth interventions post-TBI identified 12 evidence-based mHealth interventions including nine to support everyday memory (eg, Calendar app with appointments and task reminders), three to support goal attainment (eg, SMS text reminders), and three to track and manage symptoms (eg, Services Assistance Mobile and Intelligent, or SAMI, app).[47]

Several apps provide patient education to support diagnosis and risk factor management of specific types of ABI, including concussion and stroke. Other apps target specific impairments (speech, fine motor) or dysfunctions (mood, sleep) following ABI. However, there is limited evidence regarding the accuracy, evidence-basis, or efficacy of these services, making it difficult for health care providers to make informed recommendations. As a support tool, the National Health Service in England has created a database, MyTherAppy, where apps that may benefit individuals with BI are reviewed in a standardized way by trained clinical staff and patients. One validated concussion assessment tool, the King Devick sideline concussion screening, aids trained users in making recently received Food and Drug Administration approval to be used as an app, and provides another example of the broad use of mHealth applications in TBI.

Spinal cord injury

Few evidence-based mHealth interventions have been developed specifically for patients with spinal cord injury (SCI). The iMHere app is a comprehensive self-management app created and tested for individuals with spina bifida. It has been robustly researched and developed in conjunction with end user and qualified health care professionals and serves as an example of evidence-based mHealth development in rehabilitation medicine. Another example of a self-care app is SCI Health Storyline, designed to support transition patients with SCI when transitioning from inpatient care to home. Like iMHere, it includes tools for bowel and bladder management, patient education, vital sign tracking, mood and symptoms monitoring, and provider communication. However, unlike iMHere, there is little research available on this app.[48]

Several more narrowly focused apps are available that focus on a single domain of self-care, including apps to provide reminders for regularly scheduled events (catheterizations, bowel movements, pressure relief) or apps for pressure ulcer monitoring. In 2017 the Shepherd Center in Atlanta developed SCI-Ex, an activity-tracking app specific to SCI patients with descriptions of exercises recommended based on a patient's level of injury.[49] Pilot study results are forthcoming. Some activity-tracking apps in conjunction with wearable sensors (eg, Activity app with Apple Watch OS3) have started to incorporated wheelchair-based activity. This is the first step to bridge the gap in activity tracking for individuals with SCI. Numerous apps, including the Paralyzed Veterans of America app, can serve as a resource for patient education on topics related to SCI. Despite increasing interest and broadening applications, there is no current evidence behind the accuracy, development, or efficacy of the services detailed in this paragraph.

Musculoskeletal injury

Although musculoskeletal (MSK) medicine covers a broad range of diagnoses, treatment often involves activity modifications and individualized exercise programs. Several mHealth apps have been developed to supplement key aspects of MSK rehabilitation, which includes physical therapy (PT), home exercise, and patient education.

Adjunctive use of mHealth apps with traditional PT has the potential to improve patient compliance with home exercises by providing readily accessible, detailed descriptions of home exercises with multimedia support. More than 73% of patients report that they do not adhere to traditional home-exercise programs because of unclear exercise instructions.[50,51] A randomized, parallel group trial in Australia found that a PT providing home-exercise programs on an app (PhysiotherapyExercises) in combination with remote support increased adherence compared with paper handouts.[52] Many similar apps provide digital, individualized home exercise program support for PTs with patient reminders and progress reports to support adherence. In contrast, other mHealth apps provide standardized exercise programs directly to the user based on self-reported symptoms, with limited to no evidence supporting their effectiveness or safety. Providers and end users should exercise caution when using apps in lieu of, rather than in conjunction with, conventional treatment by a qualified health care professional.

Patient knowledge and understanding of their diagnoses and contributing factors affects compliance with treatment recommendations.[53] Up to 50% of patients do not understand the diagnosis or instructions provided at their medical appointments.[54] Patient-centered mHealth educational apps offer explanations of common MSK disorders, including a review of relevant anatomy and multimedia support. However, many have no research base and the validity of their content is questionable. A study evaluating 76 of the most popular apps related to orthopedic sports medicine found that most had no named medical professional involved in their development.[55] Another study found only 4 of 18 apps with a claim to prevent sports-related injuries could be supported by available literature, and five contained false claims.[56] This highlights the critical need for qualified health care involvement in the development and review of such apps before specific products are recommended.

Cardiac rehabilitation
Despite strong evidence that cardiac rehabilitation[14] is superior to counseling alone in improving the risk factors for cardiovascular disease in high-risk groups,[57,58] cardiac rehabilitation remains largely underused because of geographic availability and cost.[59,60] Adjunctive use of mHealth apps support has the potential to minimize these barriers. In a 2015 study, use of an evidence-based, guideline-driven smartphone app (Better Personal Health Assistant) in conjunction with standard cardiac rehabilitation was associated with significantly greater reductions in weight, blood pressure, rehospitalizations, and emergency department visits related to cardiovascular disease compared with cardiac rehabilitation without mHealth.[61] A 2016 RCT reported significantly greater medication adherence and overall patient satisfaction at 6-month follow-up when adding a smartphone app to usual care among 174 patients following a heart attack.[62]

Pain management
Regarding the use of mHealth apps in adult pain management, a 2014 study of 12 smartphone apps for chronic pain self-management reported that the clinical content, interface design, and usability were widely variable among apps, with limited evidence-based or guideline-driven content and little to no end user or clinician involvement in development.[63] Furthermore, most apps for pain are narrowly focused, with few supporting behavioral change or facilitating communication with medical professionals. Of 111 pain apps reviewed by Rosser and Eccleston[64] in 2011, 86% had no qualified health care involvement. These apps were categorized as providing general information (54%); facilitating symptom or medication tracking (24%); or supporting interventions for pain management, including relaxation, behavioral change, goal setting, or health care provider communication (17%), with no single app performing all three functions. In a 2013 RCT, 140 women with widespread chronic pain were provided standard care with or without an mHealth intervention (via World Wide Web app and two-way text). mHealth users had lower reported pain catastrophizing scores and more sustained improvement in functioning at 5 months, although there was high drop-out (30%). In contrast, a recent study using the pain app, Vericode, showed the app was easily introduced, well-tolerated, and had high satisfaction scores,[65]

but app use was associated with higher pain-related disability scores and lower levels of activity, despite improvement in mood.[65,66] Additional research is needed, and an emphasis on quality over quantity is key.

Amputee care

Although limited in quantity, a few narrowly focused mHealth apps are in development for patients using prostheses, largely focused on comfort and gait with lower limb prostheses. The limbWise app, developed by a PT to address common problems with the prosthesis fit, is currently undergoing efficacy testing.[67] The ReLoad app, which uses verbal instructions and music to help correct patients' gait based on sensors feedback, is also currently undergoing efficacy testing.[68] In addition, prosthetic companies have started to use mHealth apps as the control mechanism for various prostheses, allowing users to control the prosthesis without having to connect to a computer,[69] but no literature or evidence could be identified supporting the use of such products.

Applications for Community and Social Integration

Community access

Multiple crowd-sourced mapping services are now available to provide detailed community accessibility data, including standardized rating systems for entryways, hallways, bathrooms, parking, and more (eg, AXSMaps, AccessNow). Google Maps provides multiple opportunities for crowd-sourced accessibility information, such as an option for users to rate business accessibility. In May 2018, Google Maps began piloting a wheelchair-accessible route option for navigation, including sidewalk mapping to identify wheelchair-accessible sidewalk routes. In cities with robust public transit options, crowd-sourced real-time data regarding subway station accessibility are also available (eg, NYCTransit). Finally, on-demand ridesharing has become an increasing popular mode of transportation (eg, Uber, Lyft). Although the quality, availability, and timeliness of accessible services varies by location, both services offer accessible alternatives (eg, Uber WAV [wheelchair-accessible vehicle]) in select cities.

Social support

Access to support groups and peer mentors is now available digitally through dedicated apps and social media sites. Although not a substitute for face-to-face interaction, use of social media apps has been associated with self-reported improvements in social and community integration, personal growth, and illness self-management.[11,70,71] The development of special interest groups and unifying communication via social media have brought together patients and caregivers on an international level to share stories, provide support, and advocate for change.

SUMMARY

Patient-centered mHealth apps have the potential to provide multifunctional support in rehabilitation medicine, including evidence-based education, support with specific self-care tasks, tracking of biometrics and symptoms, facilitate provider-patient communication, and support comprehensive self-management. However, there are several limitations regarding the use of mHealth apps in rehabilitation medicine, including

- Limited accessibility, awareness, and training with current and emerging mHealth apps among PWD
- Limited involvement of PWD in mHealth design and usability testing

- Limited involvement of qualified rehabilitation health care providers in mHealth development and testing
- Limited number of mHealth apps grounded in evidence and few data-driven guidelines

Despite these limitations, evidence-based products are available or in development, and new products are emerging regularly. The literature and examples covered in this review highlight the current evidence, the breadth of products available and, ultimately, the need for involvement of qualified health care providers and PWD in the development and vetting of mHealth apps before recommending commercially available apps.

REFERENCES

1. Pew Research Center for Internet and Technology. Mobile fact sheet. NW Washington, DC: Inquiries D; 2017. Available at: http://www.pewinternet.org/fact-sheet/mobile/. Accessed January 21, 2019.
2. Anderson M, Perrin A. Technology use among seniors 2017. Available at: http://www.pewinternet.org/2017/05/17/technology-use-among-seniors/. Accessed March 20, 2018.
3. Research2Guidance – mHealth Economics 2017/2018: current status and future trends in mobile health. Berlin (Germany).
4. Aitken M. Patient adoption of mHealth: use, evidence and remaining barriers to mainstream acceptance. Parsippany (NJ): IMS Institute for Healthcare Informatics; 2015.
5. Mobile Medical Apps: are mobile health apps good for our health?. Available at: https://www.researchnow.com/newsroom/mobile-medical-apps-good-health-new-study-research-now-reveals-doctors-patients-say-yes-infographic/. Accessed June 2, 2018.
6. Jones M, Morris J, Deruyter F. Mobile healthcare and people with disabilities: current state and future needs. Int J Environ Res Public Health 2018;15(3) [pii:E515].
7. Anderson M, Perrin A. Disabled Americans are less likely to use technology. In: Center PR, editor 2017. Available at: http://www.pewresearch.org/fact-tank/2017/04/07/disabled-americans-are-less-likely-to-use-technology/. Accessed January 21, 2019.
8. Morris J, Jones M, Sweatman WM. Wireless technology use by people with disabilities: a national survey. J Technol Pers Disabil 2016;(4):101.
9. Morris JT, Sweatman M, Jones ML. Smartphone use and activities by people with disabilities: user survey 2016. J Technol Pers Disabil 2017;5:50–66.
10. Milne LR, Bennett CL, Ladner RE. The accessibility of mobile health sensors for blind users. J Technol Pers Disabil 2014;(2):166–75.
11. Wong D, Sinclair K, Seabrook E, et al. Smartphones as assistive technology following traumatic brain injury: a preliminary study of what helps and what hinders. Disabil Rehabil 2017;39(23):2387–94.
12. Plackett R, Thomas S, Thomas S. Professionals' views on the use of smartphone technology to support children and adolescents with memory impairment due to acquired brain injury. Disabil Rehabil Assist Technol 2017;12(3):236–43.
13. Beratarrechea A, Lee AG, Willner JM, et al. The impact of mobile health interventions on chronic disease outcomes in developing countries: a systematic review. Telemed J E Health 2014;20(1):75–82.

14. Dicianno BE, Parmanto B, Fairman AD, et al. Perspectives on the evolution of mobile (mHealth) technologies and application to rehabilitation. Phys Ther 2015; 95(3):397–405.

15. Donker T, Petrie K, Proudfoot J, et al. Smartphones for smarter delivery of mental health programs: a systematic review. J Med Internet Res 2013;15(11):e247.

16. Ernsting C, Dombrowski S, Oedekoven M, et al. Using smartphones and health apps to change and manage health behaviors: a population-based survey. J Med Internet Res 2017;19(4):e101.

17. Free C, Phillips G, Galli L, et al. The effectiveness of mobile-health technology-based health behaviour change or disease management interventions for health care consumers: a systematic review. PLoS Med 2013;10(1):e1001362.

18. Anthes E. Mental health: there's an app for that. Nature 2016;532(7597):20–3.

19. de Jongh T, Gurol-Urganci I, Vodopivec-Jamsek V, et al. Mobile phone messaging for facilitating self-management of long-term illnesses. Cochrane Database Syst Rev 2012;(12):CD007459.

20. Sundararaman LV, Edwards RR, Ross EL, et al. Integration of mobile health technology in the treatment of chronic pain: a critical review. Reg Anesth Pain Med 2017;42(4):488–98.

21. Kitsiou S, Pare G, Jaana M, et al. Effectiveness of mHealth interventions for patients with diabetes: an overview of systematic reviews. PLoS One 2017;12(3): e0173160.

22. Bell KR, Brockway JA, Hart T, et al. Scheduled telephone intervention for traumatic brain injury: a multicenter randomized controlled trial. Arch Phys Med Rehabil 2011;92(10):1552–60.

23. Bell KR, Fann JR, Brockway JA, et al. Telephone problem solving for service members with mild traumatic brain injury: a randomized, clinical trial. J Neurotrauma 2017;34(2):313–21.

24. Bell KR, Hoffman JM, Temkin NR, et al. The effect of telephone counselling on reducing post-traumatic symptoms after mild traumatic brain injury: a randomised trial. J Neurol Neurosurg Psychiatry 2008;79(11):1275–81.

25. Bell KR, Temkin NR, Esselman PC, et al. The effect of a scheduled telephone intervention on outcome after moderate to severe traumatic brain injury: a randomized trial. Arch Phys Med Rehabil 2005;86(5):851–6.

26. Bombardier CH, Bell KR, Temkin NR, et al. The efficacy of a scheduled telephone intervention for ameliorating depressive symptoms during the first year after traumatic brain injury. J Head Trauma Rehabil 2009;24(4):230–8.

27. Cikajlo I, Cizman Staba U, Vrhovac S, et al. A cloud-based virtual reality app for a novel telemindfulness service: rationale, design and feasibility evaluation. JMIR Res Protoc 2017;6(6):e108.

28. Fann JR, Bombardier CH, Vannoy S, et al. Telephone and in-person cognitive behavioral therapy for major depression after traumatic brain injury: a randomized controlled trial. J Neurotrauma 2015;32(1):45–57.

29. Ng EM, Polatajko HJ, Marziali E, et al. Telerehabilitation for addressing executive dysfunction after traumatic brain injury. Brain Inj 2013;27(5):548–64.

30. Scheenen ME, Visser-Keizer AC, de Koning ME, et al. Cognitive behavioral intervention compared to telephone counseling early after mild traumatic brain injury: a randomized trial. J Neurotrauma 2017;34(19):2713–20.

31. Vargas BB, Shepard M, Hentz JG, et al. Feasibility and accuracy of teleconcussion for acute evaluation of suspected concussion. Neurology 2017;88(16): 1580–3.

32. Vuletic S, Bell KR, Jain S, et al. Telephone problem-solving treatment improves sleep quality in service members with combat-related mild traumatic brain injury: results from a randomized clinical trial. J Head Trauma Rehabil 2016;31(2): 147–57.

33. Dicianno BE, Henderson G, Parmanto B. Design of mobile health tools to promote goal achievement in self-management tasks. JMIR Mhealth Uhealth 2017;5(7): e103.

34. Institute of Medicine Committee on the Crossing the Quality Chasm. Next steps toward a New Health Care S. In: Adams K, Greiner AC, Corrigan JM, editors. The 1st annual crossing the quality chasm summit: a focus on communities. Washington, DC: National Academies Press (US) Copyright 2004 by the National Academy of Sciences; 2004. p. 57–66. All rights reserved.

35. Fox S, Duggan M. Tracking for health 2013.

36. Lorig KR, Holman H. Self-management education: history, definition, outcomes, and mechanisms. Ann Behav Med 2003;26(1):1–7.

37. Dicianno BE, Fairman AD, McCue M, et al. Feasibility of using mobile health to promote self-management in spina bifida. Am J Phys Med Rehabil 2016;95(6): 425–37.

38. Matthew-Maich N, Harris L, Ploeg J, et al. Designing, implementing, and evaluating mobile health technologies for managing chronic conditions in older adults: a scoping review. JMIR Mhealth Uhealth 2016;4(2):e29.

39. Adult obesity causes and consequences. 2018. Available at: http://www.cdc.gov/obesity/adult/causes.html. Accessed July 2, 2018.

40. Spring B, Duncan JM, Janke EA, et al. Integrating technology into a standard weight loss treatment: a randomized controlled trial. JAMA Intern Med 2013; 173(2):105–11.

41. Oh B, Yi GH, Han MK, et al. Importance of active participation in obesity management through mobile health care programs: substudy of a randomized controlled trial. JMIR Mhealth Uhealth 2018;6(1):e2.

42. Laing BY, Mangione CM, Tseng CH, et al. Effectiveness of a smartphone application for weight loss compared with usual care in overweight primary care patients: a randomized, controlled trial. Ann Intern Med 2014;161(10 Suppl):S5–12.

43. Wang Y, Xue H, Huang Y, et al. A systematic review of application and effectiveness of mhealth interventions for obesity and diabetes treatment and self-management. Adv Nutr 2017;8(3):449–62.

44. Rivera J, McPherson A, Hamilton J, et al. Mobile apps for weight management: a scoping review. JMIR Mhealth Uhealth 2016;4(3):e87.

45. Scherer MJ. Assessing the benefits of using assistive technologies and other supports for thinking, remembering and learning. Disabil Rehabil 2005;27(13): 731–9.

46. Juengst SB, Graham KM, Pulantara IW, et al. Pilot feasibility of an mHealth system for conducting ecological momentary assessment of mood-related symptoms following traumatic brain injury. Brain Inj 2015;29(11):1351–61.

47. Juengst SB, Hart T, Sander AM, et al. Mobile health interventions after traumatic brain injuries. Current Topics in Physical Medicine & Rehabilitation Reports, in press.

48. Mortenson WB, MacGillivray MK, Sadeghi M, et al. Abstracts of scientific papers and posters at the Association of Academic Physiatrists: the usability of a self-management mobile app in inpatient rehabilitation following spinal cord injury. Am J Phys Med Rehabil 2017;96(3 Supp 1):e138–9.

49. Case A. New mobile app promotes fitness for people with spinal cord injury. Shepherd Center Newsroom; 2017. Available at: https://news.shepherd.org/new-mobile-app-promotes-fitness-for-people-with-spinal-cord-injury/. Accessed May 22, 2018.

50. Dean SG, Smith JA, Payne S, et al. Managing time: an interpretative phenomenological analysis of patients' and physiotherapists' perceptions of adherence to therapeutic exercise for low back pain. Disabil Rehabil 2005;27(11):625–36.

51. Sluijs EM, Kok GJ, van der Zee J. Correlates of exercise compliance in physical therapy. Phys Ther 1993;73(11):771–82 [discussion: 783–6].

52. Lambert TE, Harvey LA, Avdalis C, et al. An app with remote support achieves better adherence to home exercise programs than paper handouts in people with musculoskeletal conditions: a randomised trial. J Physiother 2017;63(3): 161–7.

53. Gold DT, McClung B. Approaches to patient education: emphasizing the long-term value of compliance and persistence. Am J Med 2006;119(4 Suppl 1): S32–7.

54. Atreja A, Bellam N, Levy SR. Strategies to enhance patient adherence: making it simple. MedGenMed 2005;7(1):4.

55. Wong SJ, Robertson GA, Connor KL, et al. Smartphone apps for orthopaedic sports medicine: a smart move? BMC Sports Sci Med Rehabil 2015;7:23.

56. van Mechelen DM, van Mechelen W, Verhagen EA. Sports injury prevention in your pocket?! Prevention apps assessed against the available scientific evidence: a review. Br J Sports Med 2014;48(11):878–82.

57. Balducci S, Zanuso S, Nicolucci A, et al. Effect of an intensive exercise intervention strategy on modifiable cardiovascular risk factors in subjects with type 2 diabetes mellitus: a randomized controlled trial: the Italian Diabetes and Exercise Study (IDES). Arch Intern Med 2010;170(20):1794–803.

58. Goel K, Lennon RJ, Tilbury RT, et al. Impact of cardiac rehabilitation on mortality and cardiovascular events after percutaneous coronary intervention in the community. Circulation 2011;123(21):2344–52.

59. Suaya JA, Shepard DS, Normand SL, et al. Use of cardiac rehabilitation by Medicare beneficiaries after myocardial infarction or coronary bypass surgery. Circulation 2007;116(15):1653–62.

60. Brown TM, Hernandez AF, Bittner V, et al. Predictors of cardiac rehabilitation referral in coronary artery disease patients: findings from the American Heart Association's Get With The Guidelines Program. J Am Coll Cardiol 2009;54(6): 515–21.

61. Widmer RJ, Allison TG, Lerman LO, et al. Digital health intervention as an adjunct to cardiac rehabilitation reduces cardiovascular risk factors and rehospitalizations. J Cardiovasc Transl Res 2015;8(5):283–92.

62. Johnston N, Bodegard J, Jerstrom S, et al. Effects of interactive patient smartphone support app on drug adherence and lifestyle changes in myocardial infarction patients: a randomized study. Am Heart J 2016;178:85–94.

63. Reynoldson C, Stones C, Allsop M, et al. Assessing the quality and usability of smartphone apps for pain self-management. Pain Med 2014;15(6):898–909.

64. Rosser B, Eccleston C. Mobile technology applications for pain management. J Telemed Telecare 2011;17:308–12.

65. Jamison RN, Jurcik DC, Edwards RR, et al. A pilot comparison of a smartphone app with or without 2-way messaging among chronic pain patients: who benefits from a pain app? Clin J Pain 2017;33(8):676–86.

66. Jamison RN, Mei A, Ross EL. Longitudinal trial of a smartphone pain application for chronic pain patients: predictors of compliance and satisfaction. J Telemed Telecare 2018;24(2):93–100.

67. Lee DJ. App supports self-management of prosthetic socket fit issues. The O&P Edge; 2017. Available at: https://opedge.com/Articles/ViewArticle/2017-03-02/2017-03_08. Accessed May 25, 2018.

68. Chau B. Amputee gait analysis - in a music app? iMedicalApps; 2018. Available at: https://www.imedicalapps.com/2018/04/amputee-gait-analysis-in-a-music-app/. Accessed May 25, 2018.

69. i-limb Mobile Apps. Touch Bionics by Ossur 2018. Available at: http://www.touchbionics.com/products/i-limb-mobile-apps. Accessed May 25, 2018.

70. DeHoff BA, Staten LK, Rodgers RC, et al. The role of online social support in supporting and educating parents of young children with special health care needs in the United States: a scoping review. J Med Internet Res 2016;18(12):e333.

71. Ahola Kohut S, Stinson J, Forgeron P, et al. Been there, done that: the experience of acting as a young adult mentor to adolescents living with chronic illness. J Pediatr Psychol 2017;42(9):962–9.

Moving?

Make sure your subscription moves with you!

To notify us of your new address, find your **Clinics Account Number** (located on your mailing label above your name), and contact customer service at:

Email: journalscustomerservice-usa@elsevier.com

800-654-2452 (subscribers in the U.S. & Canada)
314-447-8871 (subscribers outside of the U.S. & Canada)

Fax number: 314-447-8029

Elsevier Health Sciences Division
Subscription Customer Service
3251 Riverport Lane
Maryland Heights, MO 63043

*To ensure uninterrupted delivery of your subscription, please notify us at least 4 weeks in advance of move.

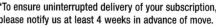
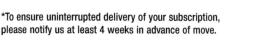

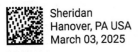
Sheridan
Hanover, PA USA
March 03, 2025